Designing Health, N̶

Gloria Gilbère, N.D., D.A.Hom., Ph.D.

Pain/Inflammation
Matters™

Foreword by
David A. Hall, M.D.
Dean Emeritus,
World Health Medical School

About the Author

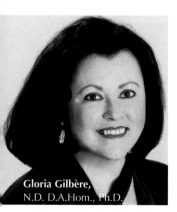

Gloria Gilbère,
N.D. D.A.Hom., Ph.D.

**Her professional
affiliations include:**

- *Member*—American Academy of Environmental Medicine
- *Member*—American Naturopathic Medical Association
- *Diplomate*— American Academy of Homeopathy
- *Board Member*— Fibromyalgia Coalition International
- *Advisory Board*— Library of Health
- *Member*—Coalition for Natural Health
- *Professor of Natural Health*— World Health Medical School
- *Member*—American Association of Nutritional Consultants
- *Digestive and Environmental Health Advisor*—Total Health magazine

Dr. Gilbère is a doctor of traditional naturopathy and natural health, and a homeopath.

She is an EcoErgonomist, environmental health consultant, health journalist and medical researcher. She consults worldwide with doctors and nutraceutical companies for product formulation and client services.

Dr. Gilbère maintains a private practice in Sandpoint, Idaho—consulting in nutritional biochemistry, detoxification, environmental health, nutrition and lifestyle modifications. She designs health plans (nationally and internationally) both via telephone consultations and at her office.

She teaches, lectures and consults worldwide, writes numerous articles for newspapers, health magazines and trade journals published in the U.S. and Canada, including: *The Doctor's Prescription for Healthy Living, Total Health, Wellness Today, Alternative Medicine, Well Being Journal, Natural Health, Natural Awakenings* (Spanish and English), *Alive & Vista* magazines (Canada only), and *Conquering the Challenge* (Newsletter of the Fibromyalgia Coalition International).

Dr. Gilbère is a keynote presenter and conducts seminars on varied disciplines of wholistic health, multiple chemical sensitivities, leaky gut and chemically-induced immune system disorders. She is internationally respected as a natural medicine researcher, environmental health consultant, and an authoritative influence in the discovery of the causes, effects, and natural solutions for leaky gut syndrome and chemically-induced immune system disorders.

Her work takes her throughout the U.S. and more than eleven countries.

As a consultant, educator, and trainer in preventive environmental health care and EcoErgonomics, her client list includes Fortune 500 companies, universities, hospitals, health care organizations, government agencies, educational facilities, corporations, and professional associations.

She has authored three previous books, listed on the facing page.

For information regarding Dr. Gilbère's consulting, speaking engagements, or interviews, CALL (360) 352-3646 (PST, 7:30 A.M. to 3:00 P.M. M-F) • FAX (208) 265-1777 • Email: info@drgloriagilbère.com • Website: www.drgloriagilbère.com

Other Books by Dr. Gloria Gilbère

I was POISONED by my body: I have a gut feeling you could be too! —*The Odyssey of a Doctor Who Reversed Fibromyalgia, Leaky Gut Syndrome and Multiple Chemical Sensitivities, Naturally.*

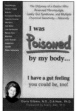

(Lucky Press, LLC: First published in 2001, 2004. Sixth printing 2005)

Invisible Illnesses: *Non-Drug Solutions to Understanding and Reversing the Common Denominators in:* • *Multiple Chemical Sensitivities* • *Fibromyalgia* • *Allergic/Inflammatory Arthritis* • *Chronic Fatigue* • *Chemically Induced Immune System Disorders* • *Leaky Gut/Irritable Bowel/Colon Disorders* • *Prescription Drug Withdrawal Syndrome*

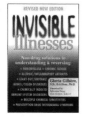

(Freedom Press: First published in 2002. Revised Edition, 2005)

Nature's Prescription Milk: *Discovering the Healing Powers of Goat-Milk Products*

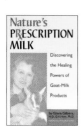

(Freedom Press, 2002)

About the "Matters" Series

The *Designing Health, Naturally* guides provide up-to-the-minute health information and vivid full-color original artwork in an easy-to-read text and format. Each book focuses on a specific natural health-related topic and explains how to improve your health and quality of life through diet, detoxification and natural time-tested healing methods.

Table of Contents

Section 1: Causes & Effects

Section 2: Heart Matters

Table of Contents

Foreword – A Doctor's Doctor

David A. Hall, M.D.

I first encountered what Dr. Gilbère labels *invisible illnesses* when I was a third-year medical student while taking a history on a hospitalized woman with severe abdominal pain. After an extensive interview, it was apparent she was severely ill. The intern in charge led me down a flight of stairs to the radiology department, grabbed the gall bladder contrast studies, and slammed them onto the reading screen. "They're normal! She's a crock!" he exclaimed. He then marched to the lady's bedside and, in an angry tone, told her she was discharged, and stormed away. I stayed with her for awhile—she was in tears, humiliated, and felt totally lost. There was something so wrong, so unjust about that scene; it stuck with me for decades as if it were yesterday.

When you go into a doctor's office, you typically receive a battery of tests. There are more abnormalities these tests don't measure than those they do—chronically ill patients don't understand this, and it is not explained. Diagnosing and treating patients with complex, chronic pain and inflammation takes time and detective work. If a practitioner uses a mindless, cookbook approach, it is destined to failure.

In the United States, we have at least two competing healthcare systems—conventional allopathic medicine and traditional natural health approaches. Relying on prescription drugs and surgery is not applicable to most chronic invisible illnesses. Many naturopathic practitioners, on the other hand, lack critical thinking and personal experience.

After practicing medicine for twenty years, I sustained an injury which evolved into an invisible illness. Receiving no help from any practitioners, I explored thousands of conventional and traditional options and research data for over ten years—there were slim-pickings. I eventually found one of Dr. Gilbère's earlier books and was struck by the rich content—things I could really use. I consulted her for advice and she provided a new valuable direction. I continue to consult with Dr. Gilbère by telephone on a regular basis and learn something new every time we speak. I have scoured the world looking for specialists on this subject—an odyssey unto itself—and no one I know comes close to Dr. Gilbère in a background of natural healing, personal experience, high energy, fund of knowledge, resourcefulness, and practical research skills.

Dr. Gilbère is a doctor's doctor; she's my doctor. When I consulted a local internist about my invisible illness years ago, he told me flat out, "I can't help you." He didn't know how, or where to refer me. Many of the large, well-known medical centers don't even recognize the existence of the invisible illnesses that Dr. Gilbère has personally recovered from, written about, and helped others design their natural path to overcome these same disorders.

The area of alternative medicine is very perplexing. You need to educate yourself and be an active participant in your own healthcare.

After working closely with Dr. Gilbère and studying her new book carefully, I can honestly testify that it belongs in the library of every person with pain, inflammation and invisible illnesses.

You are in for a real treat!

David A. Hall, M.D., Dean Emeritus
World Health Medical School
http://www.emedschool.org

Introduction

Inflammation Matters

Inflammation is the normally protective, often destructive, response of the body to infection, injury, intestinal toxic overload or the body's own tissue.

Statistical Matters

It is estimated that 26 million people, in the U.S. alone, suffer from inflammatory disorders.

As the title indicates, this volume is about assisting you in the prevention, management and reversal of pain as a result of inflammatory conditions. It's one in a series of books that are condition-specific, quick and easy, including right-to-the-point information for you and your health-care provider.

Its objective is to provide a greater understanding of known contributing factors that inhibit the body's natural repair processes.

This publication is *not* about conventional treatment—surgery or synthetic drugs to alleviate symptoms—it is about extinguishing the *fire* of inflammation from the inside out, providing time-tested tools that allow the body to build health by maximizing its own healing powers. Chronic pain and inflammation, as in fibromyalgia and arthritis for example, are known as paroxysmal conditions— the pain and inflammation come and go with flare-ups that can be debilitating. Obviously, the ideal solution is to find symptom-triggers and solutions; this book provides that, naturally.

As many of my peers have echoed before me, education is what being a doctor is all about. This book is my educational contribution for overcoming disorders I have experienced and overcome personally, and those I've observed professionally.

It's about controlling and reversing pain and inflammation through life-style, detoxification, and nutritional changes. It includes time-tested non-drug therapies and recipes for pain-free cooking and living.

CAUSE AND EFFECT

The toxic effects of NSAIDs (non-steroidal anti-inflammatory drugs) and corticosteroids are well known, especially as they relate to liver and intestinal damage. Recently, warnings have been issued regarding drugs that were heavily marketed as the "solution" to conquer most pain and inflammation…again, emphasizing the seriousness of drug side-effects.

It makes sense to learn what causes or accelerates inflammation and the accompanying pain, and then take natural measures that do not carry with them side effects that, many times, are much worse than the original condition.

WHO WILL BENEFIT FROM THIS BOOK?

Victims of arthritis, fibromyalgia, chronic fatigue, lupus, scleroderma, gout, migraine headaches, chronic generalized pain and inflammation, periodontal disease, inflammatory bowel disorders, circulatory and cardiovascular disease.

Help has arrived…this book *does not* offer quick fixes; it *does offer* proven solutions—opening the door for you to take that life-enhancing step to better health. After all, it's not quantity but quality of life that *MATTERS*, naturally.

Experience *Matters*

Chronic Inflammation, the silent killer, underscores the progression of most age-related ailments, from cardiovascular disease, and periodontal disease to obesity, not only the well-known conditions of arthritis and fibromyalgia.

Definition *Matters*

The immune system are those intelligent, highly-trained biological defenders that identify, attack and destroy disease-causing enemies.

❋ *"Healthy inflammation is akin to a small fire 'set' within a limited tissue zone to 'burn' away damaged cells and tissue debris. When inflammatory excitation is extended past the point just necessary to end the damage process, this fire can escape its normal limits. The fire is out of control and without additional effort to control it, this fire can become a chronic burn that continues for years and threatens to promote degenerative conditions of all kinds."*
—*Parris Kidd, Ph.D.*

Section 1
Causes & Effects

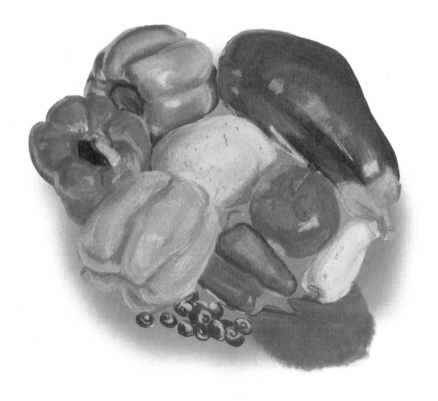

Causes & Effects

A "Shift" in View = a Renewed You

Allopathy, another term for modern conventional medicine, is based on the theory that disease is caused when the body is invaded by a foreign entity, as in a "them" or "us" mentality. When the them is defined, the treatment applied is a specific poison directed at destroying that entity, or removing it from the body, a sort of internal "ethnic cleansing"—the basis of most modern pharmacology. As long as this dominant mode exists, and all diseases are treated within the confines of this allopathic theory, there is no real hope that conventional physicians can cure chronic disorders involving pain and inflammation.

Cures will not come to those unwilling to look at underlying causes to ensure true health care verses treatments for symptom care. It is not that the allopathic approach is wrong; this approach works very well with some diseases, but not others— chronic pain from inflammation being one example.

Naturopaths and integrative physicians using other paradigms of viewing and treating generalized pain and inflammation disorders have had total success in restoring their patients to health.

INCREDIBLE FACTS—
Your entire body has the capacity to totally rebuild itself in less than 2 years, 98% of that occurs in less than 1 year…

- NEW BRAIN in 1 year
- NEW BLOOD in 4 months
- SKELETON in 3 months
- DNA in 2 months
- LIVER in 6 weeks
- SKIN in 1 month
- STOMACH lining in 5 days!

Are you still creating the same body?

Inflammation: Attack by Friendly Fire

When the immune system becomes hyperactive and malfunctions, its over-reaction produces antibodies that attack even harmless substances in the blood. This action causes formation of irritating circulating immune complexes (CICs), made up of proteins such as damaged antibodies, antigens and diseased tissues so misshapen they are foreign to the body. This process then causes the immune system to attack its own cells and tissues; the result is chronic pain and inflammation.

When CICs accumulate in the joints, for instance, they act as irritants that convert to inflammation *(See section 4 for non-drug solutions to combat CICs)*.

Most conventional treatments address symptoms of inflammation with anti-inflammatory medications, not addressing the underlying systemic cause. Yes, these medications reduce pain and inflammation and are needed for injuries and acute situations; however, they also pave a path of dangerous side effects that do nothing to start the healing process. I'm a prime example of this. My experiences after a life-threatening fall and the resulting immune system disorders from prescription drugs are discussed in detail in my book *I was POISONED by my body: The Odyssey of a Doctor Who Reversed Fibromyalgia, Leaky Gut Syndrome, and Multiple Chemical Sensitivities, Naturally*.

Furthermore, patients are not counseled on dietary changes and non-drug options, mostly because conventional medical professionals do not have the knowledge, are not interested in non-drug therapies, or simply can't take the time.

There *are* natural options to drugs, without the barrage of side effects—oftentimes worse than the original symptoms.

The non-drug solution for pain and inflammation lies in whole-food supplements, systemic oral enzymes, dietary changes, and detoxification of intestinal toxic build-up, which will be discussed later in this publication.

> ✳ *CICs = Circulating Immune Complexes. . . Over 50 million Americans suffer from some form of soft and connective tissue pain (bones, cartilaginous joints, discs, muscles, tendons, ligaments).*

Non-steroidal Anti-inflammatory Drugs (NSAIDs)

"QUICK-FIXES, DANGEROUS SIDE-EFFECTS"

In conventional medical practice, when a patient complains of pain and inflammation, the first drug widely recommended are a classification

known as non-steroidal anti-inflammatory drugs (NSAIDs). This therapy often provides effective short-term reduction of symptoms however, in the long-term, present side-effects with potentially life-altering and life-threatening complications.
I know—I'm speaking as a recovered victim.

Aspirin is widely used as a treatment for arthritis, fibromyalgia, and related conditions. The dose required is relatively high to affect lasting relief, hence toxicity often occurs—mostly tinnitus (ringing in the ears), gastric irritation, and potential intestinal bleeding.

MORE DRUGS—MORE DANGER

As aspirin becomes ineffective or intolerable, other stronger NSAIDs are often prescribed such as, but not limited to:

- Ibuprofen (Motrin, Advil, Nuprin)
- Naproxen (Naprosyn)
- Piroxican (Feldene)
- Fenoprofen (Nalfon)

As with aspirin, NSAIDs dosage must be high (as are the side effects) in order to affect relief. The most common side effect of aspirin, and other NSAIDs, is damage to the intestinal tract, leading to a potentially life-threatening disorder called leaky gut syndrome, otherwise known as toxemia or auto-intoxication (poisoning from within).

Simply stated, the walls of the intestines become porous allowing absorption of toxic matter, subsequently precipitating serious disorders such as multiple allergic response syndrome (MARS), food allergies, fibromyalgia, chronic fatigue and other chemically-induced immune system disorders.

NSAIDs provide a false sense of security from symptoms, while they cause other side effects such as inhibition of cartilage repair (collagen matrix synthesis) and, in addition, accelerate cartilage destruction. Disorders like osteoarthritis may actually manifest *accelerated symptoms* because NSAIDs *appear to suppress symptoms*, but in the process, accelerate the progression of cartilage deterioration.

According to Stephen Holt, M.D., board certified in internal medicine and gastroenterology, "NSAIDs work in arthritis by inhibiting the lipo-oxygenase conversion of lipids to prostaglandin precursors such as arachidonic acid (blocking the production of inflammatory substances in the body). This is why they're called cyclooxygenase inhibitors or COX inhibitors, for short. NSAIDs all share a potential for causing serious adverse effects, such as peptic ulceration, bleeding from the upper and lower digestive tract, damage to the liver, and the promotion of renal impairment (kidney problems), especially in the elderly."

"Boomers," the Latest Victims

According to the Centers for Disease Control and *Prevention*, the estimated cases of arthritis alone in 2005 are 21.4 million. However, because of the influx of aging baby boomers, those figures are expected to rise to 41.1 million by 2030, and that doesn't take into account all other forms of inflammatory disorders. With all the global information readily available, we boomers now have the opportunity to educate ourselves, and others, in natural options for both reversal and prevention of these life-altering disorders. After all, we're just now entering the new mid-life.

Uncommon Solution for Common Ailments

For the millions of Americans experiencing some form of joint, tendon, ligament, bone or soft-tissue discomfort, the goal is not only to find a *natural solution* for short-term relief, but also to build bone density and repair damage from the following

> ❈ *"Forty is the old age of youth. Fifty is the youth of middle-age. Sixty is the youth of old age, and seventy is when aging finally becomes an asset rather than a liability because the wisdom gained sets us free."*
> —Dr. Gloria Gilbère

disorders. This book has taken on that challenge, specifically for:

Tendonitis—An inflammation of tendons caused by repeated flexing of both tendons and muscles.

Carpal Tunnel Syndrome (CTS)—An inflammation of the nine tendons used to move the fingers, and pass from the hand to arms via a carpal tunnel in the wrist.

Bursitis—A painful inflammation of a bursa (a flat sac containing synovial fluid that facilitates the normal movement of some joints and muscles and reduces friction). Bursas are located at sites of friction, especially where tendons or muscles pass over bone. A bursa normally contains very little fluid. If injured, it becomes inflamed and may fill with fluid.

Fibromyalgia (FM)– Also known as myofascial pain syndrome, fibromyositis, or myalgic encephalomelitis (ME). A group of disorders characterized by pain and stiffness in soft tissues, including muscles, tendons (which attach muscles to bones), and ligaments (which attach bone to each other). FM is also caused by collection of toxicity in soft and connective tissues and which can result from use of medications for pain and inflammation. This can cause a condition known as leaky gut syndrome, of which I was a victim and recovered using the techniques described within as well as those discussed in my previous books.

Osteoarthritis—A chronic joint disorder characterized by degeneration of joint cartilage and adjacent bone that can cause joint pain and stiffness.

UNCOMMON COMMONALITY

In disorders like osteoarthritis and fibromyalgia specifically, the common denominators include, but are not limited to:

- Stiffness made worse by inactivity
- Generalized joint pain and stiffness
- Creaking joints
- Joint swelling
- Inflammation of soft and connective tissues
- Multiple tender spots

❋ Note: Any of the conditions to the right can trigger persistent aches, tenderness, swelling, pain, and often manifest as loss of mobility, numbness, tingling, and weakness.

Experience
Matters

Dr. Childers, through his research, proved that 74—90% of people who ache and hurt, regardless of their diagnostic "label," have a sensitivity to nightshades.

The one uncommon denominator in fibromyalgia, or the "everything hurts syndrome," is that tissues are so sensitive it feels as if the nerve endings are sitting on top of the skin. Therefore, "Don't you dare touch me!" is most commonly echoed by victims of this invisible disorder.

The Invisible Flame of Pain & Inflammation

FOODS THAT CRIPPLE

Most individuals never heard the term "nightshades," much less make the connection to a food group that ignites pain and inflammation. Nightshades are a botanical group known as *solanaceae*—making up over 92 varieties and 2,000 species.

The connection of nightshades and arthritis-type disorders was brought to the forefront largely by the efforts of Dr. Norman F. Childers, former Professor of Horticulture at Rutgers University. Dr. Childers knew first hand the agony of severe joint pain and stiffness. He discovered that after consuming a meal containing any tomatoes, he experienced severe pain. As his interest in the inflammatory responses to nightshades grew, he observed livestock kneeling in pain from inflamed joints—the livestock had consumed weeds containing a substance called *solanine*—a chemical known as an alkaloid, which can be highly toxic.

Potatoes, another nightshade, especially those stored improperly or aged, have been known to cause toxic symptoms severe enough to require hospitalization—symptoms range from gastrointestinal and general inflammation, nausea, diarrhea, and dizziness to migraines. It is believed the reason for the toxicity in potatoes is the solanine that is present in and around the green patches and the eyes that have sprouted.

Historical

Matters

The specific origin of the word "nightshade" is not clear. The English apparently called this member of the *Solanum genus* "nightshades" because of their "evil and loving" narcotic nature of the night. Also, the Latin word *"solamen"* means quieting with sedative qualities. It is written that the ancient Romans were said to prepare potions from the deadly nightshades and offer them to their enemies—they pulled the shade over their enemy's life for an eternal sleep!

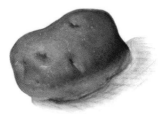

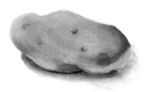

Identifying the Saboteurs

1) In L.H. Bailey's *Encyclopedia of Horticulture (1939)*, it is said, "When **potatoes** are exposed to direct sun rays and 'greened,' the deleterious substance (solanine) is so greatly increased that the water in which they are boiled is frequently used to destroy vermin on domestic animals. In any case, the water in which **potatoes** with peel are cooked should not be used in the preparation of other foods such as gravies."

2) Cholinesterase is an enzyme in the body originating from the brain that is responsible for flexibility of movement in the muscles. Solanine, present in nightshades, is a powerful inhibitor of cholinesterase. In other words, its presence can interfere with muscle movement—the cause of stiffness experienced after consuming the nightshades. All people are not sensitive to nightshades in the same degree, hence, some people develop inflammatory disorders, and others do not. However, of those already with inflammatory disorders, it is estimated over 80% experience accelerated symptoms.

3) Livestock have died in North America and Europe after ingesting potato vines, sprouts, peeling, and greened spoiled **potatoes**.

4) According to A.A. Hansen, a researcher, human fatalities of nightshades are also documented.

5) Arthritis among people in Peru is an increasingly common disease, as is the average life span of 25-30 years. Peruvians mostly grow **potatoes** instead of grain because of their climate.

6) Potatoes are used in the production of alcohol (including vodka), synthetic rubber, and starch in sizing textiles and paper. **Caution:** Do not lick envelopes, many adhesives contain potato starch.

7) Potato flour or starch is used to give body to breads, doughnuts, biscuits, candies, cookies and

Statistical *Matters*

THE COST OF PAIN
The U.S. alone spends an estimated $50 billion a year in medical expenses, lost wages and worker-compensation benefits as a result of chronic pain and inflammation representing nearly 19 million visits to doctors.

Over $20 billion a year are attributed to pain-related doctors visits. It appears our dietary lifestyle choices, which include nightshades, are a large contributing factor and one we can positively affect through life-style and dietary modifications.

soups. It is widely used in baby foods, possibly setting the stage early in life for inflammatory disorders.

8) **Paprika**, widely found in many items in grocery shelves and sprinkled on foods, comes from a non-pungent pepper mostly grown in Hungary, which may account for their higher rate of cancer than surrounding countries.

9) The **tomato** was originally known as "the love apple," and grown at first only as an ornamental. It was considered poisonous and disease-producing, and still is in some European communities. The vines and suckers are extremely poisonous to livestock as well.

10) According to *Early American Horticulture*, the tomato was known as the "cancer apple." Literature shows that the drug *tomatine* in the **tomato** has toxicity similar to solanine in the potato.

11) The **garden pepper** includes many varieties in the Capsicum family and includes **Tabasco pepper, cherry, cayenne, red cluster, bell, sweet, green, pimento, chili, long** and **red peppers. The garden pepper should not be confused with black pepper used as a condiment, which is the small berry of a tropical vine.** Black or white pepper *does not* appear to aggravate arthritis and inflammatory disorders.

12) **Eggplant** (*Solanum melongena*) was also only grown as an ornamental prior to the 20th century. It was called the "mad apple" in Mediterranean culture because it could cause insanity if eaten daily for a month. Consumption of this food aggravates inflammation and pain, the same as the other nightshades.

13) Many cultures consume **tomatillo** (*Physalis ixocarpa*) and are unaware that it is part of the nightshades; therefore the symptoms are the same as with its nightshade cousins.

14) Research warns about consuming the garden huckleberry (Solanum nigrum) native to my home in northern Idaho. Personal experience shows

NIGHTSHADE QUICK REFERENCE

✓ **Tomatoes**, all varieties (including Tomatillos)
✓ **Potatoes**, all varieties (sweet potatoes & yams are NOT nightshades)— Beware of potato starch used in many seasonings and as a thickening agent.
✓ **Peppers**, red, green, yellow, orange, jalapeno chili, cayenne, pimento
✓ **Paprika**
✓ **Eggplant**

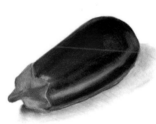

FOODS THAT CONTAIN SOLANINE although not directly in the nightshade family:

✓ **Blueberries & Huckleberries**
✓ **Okra**
✓ **Artichokes**

WHAT TO AVOID

• Homeopathic remedies containing Belladonna (known as deadly nightshade).

• Prescription and over-the-counter medications containing potato starch as a filler (especially prevalent in sleeping and muscle relaxing meds).

• Edible flowers: petunia, chalice vine, day jasmine, angel and devil's trumpets.

• Atropine and Scopolamine, used in sleeping pills

• Topical medications for pain and inflammation containing *capsicum* from cayenne pepper.

• Some vitamin C and lipoic acid can be made from potato.

CAUTION: Read labels carefully because you could be doing everything else right, and still be sabotaged by one small amount of an ingredient.

blueberries also provoke the same symptoms as the huckleberry.

15) Always be suspicious of labels reading "spices," "vegetable starch," "natural flavoring," "seasonings," "flavorings," or "seasoned salt." Most of these contain **potato starch, peppers** or **tomato** in some form. If the ingredients are not specifically listed individually, don't use it. Many sufferers have diligently adhered to their no-nightshade diet, only to experience the same symptoms from "hidden" ingredients, compounded by toxic chemical preservatives.

16) Avoid condiments such as ketchup, Worcestershire® sauce and most steak, poultry and fish sauces—instead, make them yourself so you control the ingredients.

Eating Away from Home

In our very "social" world, it's important to dine out or eat at other people's homes. I've prepared the aforementioned list for your education and that of chefs, relatives, and friends who cook and entertain for you and your family.

NEVER rely on a server to interpret *your* needs to the chef, especially if you react to nightshades as severely as my clients and I do. Ask the server to be sure to check with the chef: if he/she doesn't appear to be truly interested or informed ask to speak with the chef.

I travel extensively and have never been denied my request for accommodations—often the chef will actually come out and speak with me or send a specific message with my server. Many times, as in those regarding sauces or dressings, they've actually brought me the bottle or the recipe so I could read all the ingredients. That said, I eat in four-and five-star restaurants whenever possible because they make their food on the premises and can give me specific ingredient information, and it doesn't usually have preservatives.

Be firm, but courteous. Communicate the seriousness of your medical condition and potential reactions.

Defeat Pain & Inflammation in Twelve Weeks, Naturally

I have many clients with gastrointestinal and inflammatory disorders who resist eliminating nightshades, even for an initial trial period of twelve weeks. Those that do, however, return to report the amazing improvement in symptoms of fibromyalgia, chronic fatigue, headaches, arthritis, gout, carpal tunnel, irritable bowel and scleroderma, to name a few—after all, the only thing you have to lose is your discomfort!

Chapter 3 of this book is provided specifically to give you the benefit of the nightshade-free gourmet recipes that I created, and also, hopefully, to inspire you to create your own. Enjoy!

✤ *Addicted to Nightshades???*
It has been suggested by people who comment, I cannot do without tomatoes or potatoes," that they may be just as addicted to this specific group of foods as those addicted to tobacco, also a nightshade. Someday scientists may actually find and validate evidence that nightshade foods are as addicting as their tobacco cousin.

Section 2
Heart

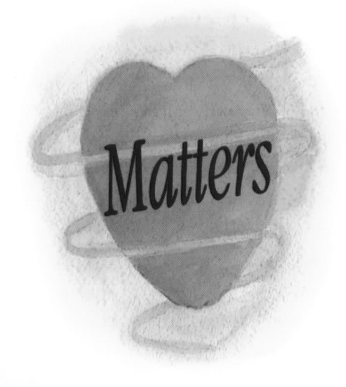

Heart Matters

A Killer of Epidemic Proportions

Heart disease has become an epidemic killer, especially for those of us baby boomers at such high risk due to our age and "modern" lifestyles. Therefore, I'm including extensive research, solutions and comments within this book. When you add to the risk factors for heart disease all the components of Syndrome "X" (also known as the baby boomer or metabolic syndrome), including pain and inflammation, we must stand-up, pay attention, and take action because the following facts can no longer be ignored:

- Every 20 seconds, someone in the U.S. has a heart attack.
- One in five Americans has high blood pressure.
- Cardiovascular disease has been the number one killer in the U.S. every year since 1900, (except for 1918, due to an epidemic of influenza and WWI).
- Close to 6 million hospitalizations in the U.S. each year are due to some form of cardiovascular disease.
- One hundred million Americans have elevated blood cholesterol; 65 million have borderline cholesterol levels between 200-239 mg/dl.
- Sedentary individuals are twice as likely to have a heart attack as those who exercise regularly.
- 700,000 Americans suffer a stroke each year.

Research Matters

According to the *Journal of the American Medical Association (JAMA)*, a seven-year study of 20,525 women showed that even among those with very low initial blood pressure, high levels of CRP were associated with an increased risk of developing hypertension. Women with the highest levels of CRP measured at the beginning of the study were about twice as likely to develop hypertension.

The Link Between Inflammation & Heart Disease

Recent research shows, without a doubt, that cardiovascular disease is linked to inflammation. Researchers suggest that the body sees plaque accumulation in the arteries as an assault or injury to the walls of the blood vessel, leading to white cells attacking and inflaming the plaque. As this occurs, it causes a breakdown, creates a blood clot that blocks blood flow, and subsequently induces a heart attack.

Normally, inflammation is a sign that the immune system is in high gear, increasing production of cytokines (proteins that attack germs and repair damaged tissue). Inflammation should subside once an area has healed; *when it does* not, serious problems can occur. A study conducted at Tufts University in Massachusetts found that an increase in inflammatory proteins was associated with loss of mobility, muscle strength, and the ability to fight disease.

Measuring Inflammation

A reliable measure of inflammation is performed by a test that measures C-reactive protein (CRP). CRP is a special type of protein produced by the liver that is *only present during episodes of acute inflammation*. This is not an inflammatory specific test; however, it does give a general indication of acute inflammation. Physicians use this test to check for rheumatoid arthritis or rheumatic fever flare-ups and it is also helpful in monitoring response to various healing modalities.

The measurement of CRP is easy and affordable through your health care provider. It is a simple blood test that is analyzed by a medical laboratory through a traditional blood-draw.

Heart Attack Markers

Recent studies suggest a connection between heart attacks and elevated C-reactive proteins. Many consider CRP levels to be a positive risk factor for coronary artery disease.

Inflammation Matters

In instances of rheumatic inflammation as in rheumatoid arthritis and systemic lupus erthematosus, the CRP levels do not always show as elevated—the reason for this is not yet known, however, what is known is that a low level of CRP does not mean there is no inflammation.

Keep in mind that any type of inflammation will elevate the CRP level in the blood. The following are examples of CRP elevations *not* necessarily *heart related*:

- Pneumonia—40 to 50
- Chronic Arthritis/Fibromyalgia—10 to 30
- Low-grade inflammation—1 to 6
  Note: In the past, laboratory tests only measured levels greater than 6. Now there is a new high-sensitivity CRP test, also known as the "cardio" CRP that measures levels between 1 and 6. Because we now know that ischemic* cardiovascular disease is believed to be an inflammatory disease, it's more important than ever to know your levels of CRPs to assess risk factors for coronary artery disease. The levels between 1 and 6 are divided into three categories:
- Below 1: lowest risk
- 1 to below 3: intermediate risk
- 3 or more: high risk

CRP FLUCTUATIONS

C-reactive protein levels can fluctuate from day to day due to the following:

- Aging
- High blood pressure
- Smoking
- Chronic fatigue
- Inactivity (sedentary life)
- Lack of Sleep
- Estrogen (HRT)
- Insulin resistance
- Clinical depression
- Alcohol

*The term **ischemic** means that an organ, in this case the heart muscle, has not received enough blood and oxygen. In a condition known as Cardiomyopathy, a ischemic disease, the term "cardio" refers to the heart and "myopathy" means this is a muscle-related disease.

Elevated CRP: Risk Factors

Keep in mind that in a healthy body, there should be no CRP present in blood serum.

When the CRP markers are high, it can indicate the following conditions or high risk factors, but not limited to:

- Pneumococcal pneumonia
- Rheumatoid arthritis
- Rheumatic fever
- Fibromyalgia
- Cancer
- Tuberculosis
- Myocardial infarction (heart attack)
- Lupus
- Inflammatory bowel disease

Note: Positive CRP results can occur during the last half of pregnancy or with the use of oral contraceptives. (Information provided by Lisa Christopher, M.D., Division of Rheumatology, Johns Hopkins Hospital, Baltimore, MD. Review provided by VeriMed Healthcare Network.)

Statistical Matters

The American Heart Association, the U.S. Centers for Disease Control and *Prevention Magazine* recently endorsed CRP testing for people with even a moderate risk of heart disease.

Everyday, nearly 1,400 women die from heart disease!

Getting to the Heart of It, Naturally!

Conventional prescription drugs are necessary when an acute or life-threatening situation exists. In contrast, however, there are safe, natural ingredients that, in many cases, have the same or better overall health effects—without drug side effects.

This section will discuss some of the best-researched and applied non-drug solutions to preventing and reversing inflammation and the resulting cardiovascular diseases.

Statistics Matter

Heart disease kills more women under 45 than any other single disease.

- **Hawthorn (*Crateagus oxyacantha*)** This herb strengthens cardiovascular function on many levels, one being through its composition of bioflavonoids. Bioflavonoids protect the circulatory system by reducing cholesterol and atherosclerotic plaque, as well as decreasing the permeability of capillaries and other blood vessels. Hawthorn is a natural vasodilator (a substance that relaxes and dilates the blood vessels, allowing increased blood flow). Researchers have also found hawthorn to improve oxygen intake—benefiting overall circulation and blood flow, and reducing stress to the heart. Hawthorne is used in many herbal and homeopathic complexes like Cardiogenics® and a unique liquid herbal blend called Heart Matters™ (see resource guide).

- **Rutozym™ (*Systemic enzyme formula*)** This unique blend of proteolytic enzymes, including bromelain (from pineapple) and papain (from papaya), are known to effectively rebalance the body's inflammatory responses. It is enhanced with rutin to strengthen capillaries and connective tissue, and contains "nature's aspirin," white willow bark. Rutozym is *not* designed as a digestive enzyme blend, but rather a bloodstream blend to counteract the health factors known to affect heart health, including lowering CRP levels. Details regarding the health benefits of Rutozym are listed later in this section.

Circulation, Anti-aging & Health, Naturally

We already know that inflammation is the major underlying cause of heart disease; inflammation damages blood vessels. Once that happens, the nutrients from the blood begin to leak through the

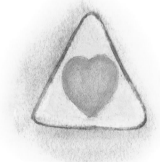

vessel wall (much the same as the inflammation and leakage that occur in leaky gut syndrome from the intestines) and can cause localized swelling and skin blotching.

The main function of the blood is to deliver nutrients and oxygen to tissues in the body, including the skin. Since skin, hair and nails are at the end of the food chain, it is absolutely essential the nutrients they require are properly delivered through a vigorous blood flow throughout the body.

Rutin to the Rescue

A bioflavonoid called rutin, promotes heart health for certain, but also benefits skin. Rutin has been used in natural medicine for centuries because of its ability to strengthen blood vessel walls and control permeability (leaking). This enables circulating blood to deliver the precious nutrients to all parts of the body equally, including the skin. In addition, rutin is also a potent antioxidant and fights free radicals. Rutin is found as part of a complex in the product previously mentioned called Rutozym™, discussed elsewhere in this chapter.

Statistics
Matter
In the U.S. alone, over 600,000 hospitalizations for DVT occur annually, of those 200,000 end in death.

Avoiding Blood Clots, Naturally

Okay, so we know that every 34 seconds heart disease claims another American life. What most of us do not know is that blood clots, specifically known as Deep Venous Thrombosis (DVT) or Thrombophlebitis, occur in approximately one out of every 20 people over a lifetime, including this author.

According to legend, a warrior named Minamoto Yoshiie found and tasted boiled soybeans that had been left on straw and had fermented. As far as history shows, that was the initial discovery of *natto*. It is believed that by the end of the Edo period (1603 to 1867), *natto* had become a regular part of Japanese cuisine in many areas.

I can, unfortunately, speak from experience after being a victim of DVT which became a life-threatening pulmonary embolism after my much-written-about accident and the subsequent book that describes my odyssey in *I Was POISONED by My Body*.

Blood clots are nothing to take lightly. The best common description of blood clots is given by Dr. Donald Schreiber, M.D., C.M. Assistant Professor of Surgery, Stanford University School of Medicine… "The development of venous thrombosis is best understood as the activation of coagulation in areas of reduced flood flow. This explains why the most successful prophylactic regimens are anti-coagulation and minimizing venous stasis." In other words, the best insurance against blood clots is to keep the blood flowing.

That said, I was constantly researching for natural substances to keep the blood from clotting, as well as to prevent heart disease.

"Nat" to Worry. There is a Natural Solution.

There is a food-based substance that most North Americans know little of—natto.

Natto is a fermented soy-based cheese, common in Japanese culture for over 2000 years. It's sticky, odorous nature demands an acquired taste for most westerners.

Some twenty-three years ago, a doctor by the name of Hiroyuki Sumi discovered the important clot-dissolving nature of natto. Dr. Sumi was a researcher at Chicago University Medical School, studying physiological chemistry.

Dr. Sumi's passions included identifying natural ingredients that dissolve thrombi (clots), and non-drug preventative and curative therapies for heart attacks, strokes, senility, and sudden death. Finally, his persistence paid high dividends. After examining more than 170 natural foods, he discovered that the fibrin (the material that causes platelets to stick together and cause clots) completely dissolved within eighteen hours of being exposed to natto. Eventually, Dr. Sumi isolated the actual active ingredient in natto, a fibrinolytic enzyme*, which he named "nattokinase."

According to Dr. Sumi, nattokinase shows *"potency matched by no other enzyme."* Since his original discovery, clinical findings validate that nattokinase is an extremely potent and safe fibrinolytic enzyme.

HEALTH PIONEERS

Through the work started by Dr. Karl Ransberger in Germany, a product was developed that included nattokinase and two systemic enzymes used in the world's most widely researched enzyme blend, Wobenzym N™. These two systemic enzymes have shown to be effective in normalizing inflammation, but that wasn't enough. The new formula, Rutozym™ not only improved blood flow; it strengthened the integrity of blood vessels and helped manage the body's systemic inflammatory response – promoting better overall health.

Rutozym™ works by reinforcing your body's own enzymes—the building blocks of life that are responsible for every chemical action in the body. Rutozym™ is a plant-based systemic enzyme formula containing nattokinase. In addition, it contains other carefully blended ingredients like proteolytic enzymes bromelain and papain, known to effectively rebalance inflammatory responses. Rutin is also included because it strengthens capillaries and connective tissue. Last, but certainly not least, the formula includes white willow bark, known as "nature's aspirin."

Fermentation *Matters*

During fermentation, vitamins B_2, K and minerals such as iron, calcium, and potassium are created. In addition, the enzymes contained in *natto* aid digestion, along with the bonus these enzymes provide for dissolving blood clots.

Rutozym™ *Matters*

- Manages age-related protein accumulation
- Naturally pacifies inflammatory responses
- Enteric coating makes it pH resistant and better utilized
- Rids the body of cross-linked fibrin
- Strengthens vessel wall integrity

* breaks down fibrin and provides antioxidant activity

> ✳ *"Antioxidants act as metabolic regulators, antitoxins and anti-inflammatories. These miraculous nutritional ingredients are imperative fortifiers of our immune systems as well as powerful therapy and co-therapy in confronting the degenerative diseases that invade our organ systems."*
> *—Parris M. Kidd, Ph.D., Scientific Advisor, Total Health magazine)*

I find that taking two Rutozym™ tablets twice daily is sufficient for my overall circulation and as insurance for cardio health. That said, when I travel, especially by air, I take six a day to further reduce my risk of again developing blood clots from lack of movement and being in a pressurized aircraft.

Anti-oxidants: A Chain is only as Strong as its Weakest Link

As the quote to the left emphasizes, no matter what other nutritional intervention, we must also supplement with antioxidants in order for the entire healing processes to work in synchronicity and have effective long term results.

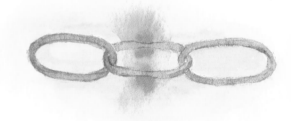

Free Radicals: Guilty as Charged

It's been said that free radicals, and the damage they cause, are the silent terrorists that infiltrate our body and alter the metabolic consciousness to that of attack and destroy.

What are the consequences of free radicals? They are basically responsible for the creation or contribution to the following conditions: heart disease, fibromyalgia, arthritis, alzheimer's, parkinson's, age-related wrinkles and aging in general. We don't have a large amount of input as to the external toxins we're exposed to; however, we do have the ability to supplement with quality nutrient antioxidants to build our wall of defense and neutralize free radicals. Oxygen-based life-forms cannot exist without antioxidants—they are the body's protectors.

THE GREAT DEFENDER

Stephen Sinatra, M.D., a respected cardiologist, reported that much of the heart disease he observes in women has been directly linked to Coenzyme Q_{10} (CoQ_{10}) deficiency. More than 100 clinical studies document the benefits of CoQ_{10} for the following conditions:

- Cardiomyopathy
- Heart failure
- Angina
- Hypertension

CoQ_{10} is a fairly new nutrient to conventional medicine, but not to science. The scientific community has known it as ubiquinone, first isolated by Dr. Frederick Crane and his associates at the Enzyme Institute of the University of Wisconsin in 1957. The most important discovery by Dr. Crane is that CoQ_{10} controls the flow of oxygen within individual cells.

CoQ_{10} is a biochemical found in such foods as beef, sardines, spinach, and peanuts; interestingly, most humans are extremely deficient. It is a natural, fat-soluble nutrient present in virtually all cells and vital to the production of adenosine triphosphate (ATP), the energy-rich compound used for all energy-requiring processes in the body.

Definition

Matters

"CoQ_{10} is an essential nutrient that supplies the biochemical 'spark' that creates cellular energy. Without it, various mechanisms in the body quickly begin to fail, exposing us to a host of major medical problems." —Dr. Emile G. Bliznakov, President and Scientific Director, Lupus Research Institute.

❋ *If CoQ_{10} is oil-based, it is better absorbed if taken with a little fat or oil. If it is water-soluble, it is well absorbed taken any time.*

CoQ$_{10}$ Benefits
Matter

- Improves the heart's pumping ability
- Improves blood circulation
- Increases tolerance to exercise
- Improves heart muscle-tone
- It crosses the blood-brain barrier for entry into the mitochondria*, facilitating the ability to make ATP
* See "Heart Talk Matters"

AUTHOR'S RECOMMENDATION
CoQ$_{10}$ deficiency also shows as a potential contributor to some cancers, particularly in women. The recommended daily amount is 50 to 200 mg. depending on specific risk factors. I personally take 200 mg. daily. See resource guide for a quality supplier.

Health
Matters

Each cigarette smoked eliminates 25mg from the body's Vitamin C cache.

A Life Saved, A Lesson Learned

A patient in her early fifties was diagnosed with the condition of a rapidly degenerating heart function. Her physician gave her no more hope than surviving a couple of weeks.

Several years later, she is alive and well, her heart strong, and she's remarkably active. This woman was a participant in a study at the Hospital of Rehabilitation in Bornheim-Merten, West Germany. She was so desperately ill that her cardiac output (the total volume of blood being pumped from the heart) had dropped to life-threatening levels. Conventional medications like digitalis, beta-blockers, and vasodilators had no beneficial effect. CoQ$_{10}$ supplementation was then added to her diet. *Within five weeks*, her cardiac output rose to the point where her heart was again pumping a healthy amount of blood (4.5 liters per minute)—a life saved, a lesson learned.

Additional Heart Protectors

The following "heart protectors" should also be considered:

- **Garlic**—Garlic reduces free-radical damage, breaking-down cholesterol and inhibiting infiltration of damaged fats and cholesterol through the walls of our arteries. It lowers cholesterol, triglycerides, blood pressure and keeps platelets from forming dangerous clots. *Note:* I take a daily supplement named Garlic 7000™. It has been a huge factor in assisting me to lower my cholesterol and keep my blood clotting time at a healthy level. Having been a victim of life-threatening blood clots, garlic in addition to Rutozym™ are two of the most important supplements I consume to ensure healthy blood flow. The garlic is tasteless and odorless; however, it does have a strong odor when the bottle is opened. See resource guide.

- **Vitamin E**—The fat-soluble antioxidant that everyone needs. Start slowly with 100 IUs and build up to 400 to 800 per day under the guidance of your health-care provider. D-alpha tocopherol or mixed tocopherols are best. For best absorption, take with a meal containing fat.
- **Magnesium**—An important mineral that most either ignore or forget about. It is the number one mineral Americans are deficient in. It is one of the most important nutrients for heart health. Take 400 to 600 mg. per day with meals. If you experience loose stools, reduce the amount until normal elimination is achieved and continue at that level (Listen to your body, it provides specific signals).
- **Vitamin C**—One of the most powerful antioxidants also increases interferon production and is a potent stimulator of T-effector cell activity. It reduces lipid production in the brain and spinal cord from free-radical damage by crossing the blood-brain barrier. *It protects after toxic chemical exposures by increasing natural killer cell activity and B-cell function.*

I recommend 2,500 to 4,000 mg. per adult, to bowel tolerance*, particularly for individuals with disorders discussed in this book.

Heart Statistics *Matter*

- Each day, the heart propels 2,000 gallons of blood through 65,000 miles of blood vessels by beating 100,000 times.
- Heart cells have a greater number of mitochondria, subsequently requiring more CoQ_{10} than any other cell. Each heart cell can have thousands of mitochondria to meet energy demands.

Statistical *Matters*

The National Institutes of Health, Bethesda, Maryland, reported that only 9% of Americans have optimal Vitamin C levels.

* until loose stools are experienced

Heart Talk

Matters

Clot—A clot is formed when platelets and circulation substances in the blood stick together. A clot can block or reduce blood flow.

DVT—Deep Venous Thrombosis (blood clots)

Heart Attack—A heart attack occurs when one or more coronary arteries supplying blood to the heart are partially or fully blocked.

Plaque—When cholesterol and other cellular debris stick to the walls of the arteries. Plaques can break and start the platelets to aggregate.

Platelets—Platelets are a type of blood cells, and are typically like very small particles. They play an important role in blood clotting and are sometimes also called thrombocytes.

Platelet Aggregation—Indicates clumping of platelets. In healthy individuals, platelet aggregation plugs a small hole in a damaged blood vessel.

Ischemic Stroke—A clot blocks blood flow in the artery leading to the brain.

continued on next page

Warning Signs of a Heart Attack

The American Heart Association warns that not all heart attacks are sudden. I mention this so you don't become complacent when symptoms start slowly with mild discomfort or pain. Please read the following symptoms until you know them inside-out, it could save your life and that of a loved one.

HEART ATTACK

- **Chest discomfort**—most heart attacks involve discomfort in the center of the chest that lasts more than a few minutes, or discomfort that goes away and comes back. It can feel like uncomfortable pressure, squeezing, fullness or pain. Note: The pain is very different from that of an inflamed liver, which causes fullness and pain on the right side under the breast that can extend to beneath the left breast as if a swelling that follows a woman's bra line.
- **Discomfort in other areas of the upper body** include:
  - pain or discomfort in one or both arms
  - in the back
  - in the neck
  - in the jaw (not a TMJ type pain)
  - in the stomach (not indigestion from lack of enzymes)
- **Shortness of breath**, especially chest discomfort before chest pain emerges.
- **Other signs** are:
  - breaking-out in a cold sweat for no apparent reason
  - nausea
  - light-headedness

STROKE

- Sudden numbness or weakness of the face, arm or leg, especially on one side of the body
- Sudden confusion, trouble speaking or understanding
- Sudden trouble seeing in one or both eyes
- Sudden trouble walking, dizziness, loss of balance or coordination
- Sudden, severe headache with no apparent reason

CARDIAC ARREST

Cardiac Arrest strikes sudden and without warning.

- Sudden loss of responsiveness, no response to gentle shaking
- No normal breathing, victim does not take a normal breath for several seconds
- No signs of circulation, movement or coughing

Heart Talk
Matters continued

Stroke—When blood flow through an artery supplying blood to the brain is significantly reduced or blocked. As a result, the brain is temporarily or permanently damaged. Stroke is also called a cerebrovascular accident.

Hemorrhagic Stroke—Occurs when a blood vessel ruptures, causing blood to leak into the brain.

Mitochondria—Highly specialized structures within each cell that are often referred to as cell powerhouses. These tiny energy-producers produce 95% of the energy the body requires, especially the heart. A cells' ATP production is dependent on adequate amounts of CoQ_{10}.

AUTHOR'S NOTE
Everything else you do for health is irrelevant if you don't take care of the "heart" of the body's operating system, naturally.

Section 3
Nightshade-FREE Recipes

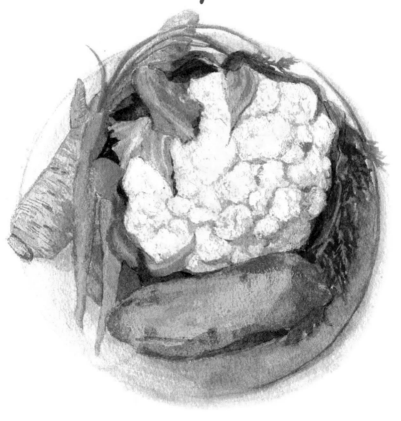

Conversion *Matters*

Liquid Weights		Dry Weights		Temperatures	
U.S. *Measurements*	*Metric* *Equivalents*	*U.S.* *Measurements*	*Metric* *Equivalents*	*Fahrenheit*	*Celcius* *(Centigrade)*
1/4 teaspoon	1.23 ml	1/4 ounce	7 grams	32°F (water freezes)	0°C
1/2 teaspoon	2.5 ml	1/3 ounce	10 grams	200°F	95°C
3/4 teaspoon	3.7 ml	1/2 ounce	14 grams	212°F (water boils)	100°C
1 teaspoon	5 ml	1 ounce	28 grams	250°F	120°C
1 dessert spoon	10 ml	1 1/2 ounces	42 grams	275°F	135°C
1 tablespoon (3 teaspoons)	15 ml	1 3/4 ounces	50 grams	300°F (slow oven)	150°C
		2 ounces	57 grams	325°F	160°C
2 tablespoons (1 ounce)	30 ml	3 ounces	85 grams	350°F (moderate oven)	175°C
		3 1/2 ounces	100 grams	375°F	190°C
1/4 cup	60 ml	4 ounces (1/4 pound)	114 grams	400°F (hot oven)	205°C
1/3 cup	80 ml			425°F	220°C
1/2 cup	120 ml	6 ounces	170 grams	450°F (very hot oven)	230°C
2/3 cup	160 ml	8 ounces (1/2 pound)	227 grams	475°F	245°C
3/4 cup	180 ml			500°F	260°C
1 cup (8 ounces)	240 ml	9 ounces	250 grams	(extremely hot oven)	
2 cups (1 pint)	480 ml	16 ounces (1 pound)	464 grams		
3 cups	720 ml				
4 cups (1 quart)	1 liter			**Approximate Equivalents**	
4 quarts (1 gallon)	3 3/4 liters			1 kilo is slightly more than 2 pounds	
				1 liter is slightly more than 1 quart	

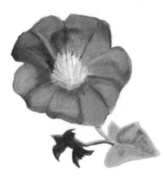

Cooking to Combat Pain & Inflammation

In recommending any type of elimination diet, there is always resistance—echoing, "It's too difficult to find adequate substitutions." When people have tried every other means to eliminate the pain and stiffness that deteriorates their quality of life, to no avail, they finally agree to eliminate the nightshade family of foods. The most challenging aspect of the diet is to take time to read labels. Many of the nightshades are actually hidden in a wide variety of prepared foods, supplements and medications. Therefore, if you don't take time to *scrutinize every label before buying or eating* its contents, you will not achieve the benefits.

Initial Elimination Challenge

Many sufferers follow the elimination diet for twelve weeks, only to claim their symptoms are not relieved after having consumed hidden sources of nightshades unsuspectingly. For maximum health benefits, the recommended time to be completely without food from the nightshade family is twelve weeks. If after that time you do not feel relief, reintroduce your favorite food from the nightshade family every day for one week. Notice how you feel; pay special attention to any added stiffness, pain, aches or loss of energy, be honest with yourself. When you learn to genuinely listen to your body, it will never betray you.

A Doctor's Perspective

I knew giving up potatoes was going to be a hardy sacrifice, mashed potatoes have been my comfort food since childhood. In searching for alternatives, I

Beware of . . .

EDIBLE FLOWERS
The nightshade plants are not limited to those we eat or smoke. Ornamental plants are also in the family: petunia, chalice vine, day jasmine, and the angel's and devil's trumpets. Other plants have long provided medicinal drugs such as belladonna, atropine and scopolamine (used widely as an ingredient in sleeping pills).

Beware of . . .

...foods fried in oil where nightshades have been cooked, i.e. fish cooked in the same oil as french fries. Also, foods like lobster could be boiled in water potatoes were cooked in.

found using parsnips just as satisfying. I peel them, boil them, mash them, slice them and sauté them with onions like hash-brown potatoes. I include them in oven roasting and even make fried mashed parsnip patties from leftovers. The taste is sweeter but pleasant, and most importantly, does not cause the pain and inflammation that last for days and even weeks from consuming nightshades.

Beware of Some Medications & Homeopathics

Another consideration is to refrain from taking any homeopathic remedies that contain belladonna (known as the deadly nightshade). Belladonna is widely used in homeopathy with positive results for varied conditions. However, anyone sensitive to the nightshades, should refrain from any remedy containing this substance.

A hidden source of nightshades is also contained in many prescription and over-the-counter medications. For instance, some sleeping and muscle relaxing medications contain potato starch as filler. They may assist in helping you sleep and, in addition, add to your pain for days to come, without ever recognizing the source of your discomfort. In the event you need to take a prescription medication, be sure to ask the pharmacist about the ingredients and tell him/her that you do not want any prescription with added fillers that contain nightshades.

Topical medications for pain and inflammation are another source of concern. Many companies are marketing creams and ointments that contain capsicum (the substance contained in cayenne pepper). Read all labels carefully.

✳ Sweetpotatoes and yams are NOT nightshades.

Beware of...

...anything containing modified food starch, potato starch, modified vegetable protein (MVP) or hydrolyzed vegetable protein (HVP), they either contain nightshades or dangerous preservatives that do not specifically have to be disclosed.

What You Eat Matters

The following recipes are just a "taste" of what can be accomplished when you become determined to regain a quality and taste of life you grew to expect. Being a gourmet cook gave me a huge advantage in creating tasty recipes that do not ignite the flame of inflammation—stealing quality of life from its victims, including my own. Countless readers and clients have been asking for my nightshade-free cooking sensations, here's a start.

INSTEAD OF POTATOES

Mock Potato Casserole

2 yams or sweet potatoes
2 Walla Walla or Maui sweet onions
3 parsnips
1/3 cup chopped parsley
1 cup heavy cream *
2 garlic cloves (minced) or 2 shallots
1/4 cup goat cheese
1 carrot

A unique taste that can be altered to suit your palette and is a great substitute for scalloped potatoes.

Peel and thinly slice yams, onions, garlic, carrot and parsnips. Bake on cooking sheet for 30 minutes at 325°F. Use a greased casserole dish (or use parchment paper) to layer the baked vegetables with cream, salt/pepper and goat cheese. Return to the oven and bake an additional 45 minutes at 325°F.

Options—Sprinkle shredded cheese and parsley on top before serving.

*If using milk substitute, thicken with 1 or 2 T of either rice or tapioca flour. You can also thicken with arrowroot if you have sensitivities to either of the above.

*If you cannot tolerate cheese but can tolerate cream or yogurt, you may substitute for the cheese.

Mashed Creamy Caultatos

Be sure to steam the cauliflower and garlic, until soft, for approx. 15 minutes; drain. In a food processor or blender, add cauliflower, garlic, mayo/ranch dressing and salt. Blend until creamy.

Options—You can garnish with chopped fresh parsley, black or white pepper, or a bit of finely shredded organic goat cheese. If dairy isn't a health challenge, you can sprinkle some grated organic sharp cheddar cheese and organic butter.

6 cups cauliflower florets (not the stems)
1 1/2 qts. water (approx.)
2 cloves garlic, chopped fine (optional)
1/4 cup ranch dressing or Best Foods real mayonnaise
1/8 tsp salt
Organic butter

> ✳ *Cauliflower is an excellent source of vitamin C, and a good source of folacin and potassium.*

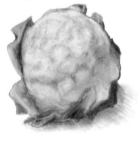

Barely Barley Taters

This recipe is quite unique, and makes a wonderful substitute for potatoes or rice if you happen to be sensitive to those ingredients.

Melt butter or coconut oil in frying pan.
Add onion, mushrooms and barley.
Sauté until lightly browned taking care not to burn.
Place into a 1 1/2 quart casserole.
Add almonds, green onions, chicken broth, season to taste, and stir into the other ingredients in casserole.
Cover and bake at 350ºF for about 1 1/2 hours until barley is soft and tender.
SERVES 6 TO 8

1 cup pearl barley
1/3 cup thinly sliced almonds or pecans
1/3 cup diced green onions
1 cup (approx.) low salt chicken broth
1/2 cup sliced fresh mushrooms (if fungi are allowed in your diet)
1 cup finely chopped onion
White or black pepper to taste
Organic butter or extra-virgin coconut oil (approx. 1 T)

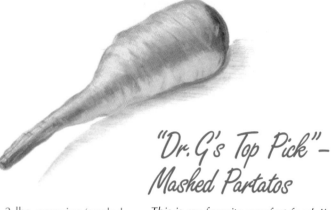

"Dr. G's Top Pick" – Mashed Partatos

2 lbs. parsnips (peeled and cut into cubes)
2 T organic butter or coconut oil
Pinch of salt
Dash of pepper
1/4 cup goat's milk, rice milk, or heavy cream (warmed)
3 fresh garlic cloves (finely chopped) "optional"
Finely chopped parsley as desired
Fresh goat, sharp cheddar or parmesan cheese (optional)

This is my favorite comfort food. I've served them for a formal holiday dinner and received rave reviews. Some of my male guests were hesitant that a nightshade-free turkey dinner wouldn't be as tasty or satisfying. As history has shown at my house, the partatos were the first thing to disappear with comments like "What in the heck is in this, they're delicious?" If male guests offer that type of positive response, you know you have a winning recipe.

Scrub, rinse and peel parsnips, retain the peelings and add to cooking water.

Cut the peeled parsnips into small pieces and cook for approx. 20 minutes until soft enough to mash easily. Drain and mask with a potato masher or preferably an electric mixer to get a softer texture. (Cook them the same as you would potatoes.)

Add butter or coconut oil.

Gradually add the warmed milk or cream, chopped garlic, parsley, cheese and continue to beat until fluffy. If the mixture needs thinning, or you need to reduce milk content, add some of the parsnip water instead of more milk or cream.

If you are not dairy sensitive, this dish is delicious with grated parmesan or Romano cheese and an additional dollop of organic butter. Once you repair your digestive system, you can generally indulge occasionally in additional ingredients, get creative.

Partato Pancakes

These little patties are delicious for breakfast served with eggs and your favorite nightshade-free hollandaise sauce or gravy. They are also excellent served warm with a dollop of fresh sour cream, apple or plum sauce or goats' cheese—a great starch replacement for rice or pasta.

2 T very finely chopped onion
1 T organic butter or coconut oil
2 cups *chilled* mashed partatos *(see recipe page 44)*
1 egg, slightly beaten
1/4 cup rice or tapioca flour (on flat plate)

In a large skillet, cook onion in butter or coconut oil.

Drain oil from onion (reserve oil and drippings).

In a large bowl, combine onion, chilled mashed partatos and egg.

Shape into six 3-inch patties.

Gently dip both sides of patty into flour on flat plate.

Add any remaining oil or drippings to skillet or add more to brown the patties.

Heat over medium heat until patties get a thin golden "skin."

SERVES 6 (or as many patties as your mixture makes)

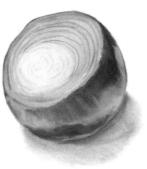

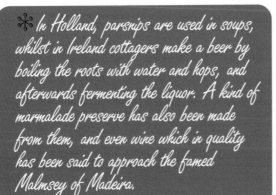

❊ In Holland, parsnips are used in soups, whilst in Ireland cottagers make a beer by boiling the roots with water and hops, and afterwards fermenting the liquor. A kind of marmalade preserve has also been made from them, and even wine which in quality has been said to approach the famed Malmsey of Madeira.

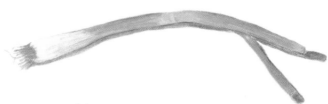

Hash Browned Partatos

Approx. 6 large
 parsnips
3 T butter or
 coconut oil
¼ cup finely chopped
 onion or green onion
Dash of salt and pepper

Wash, peel and shred parsnips.

Warm a large skillet and add butter or coconut oil

In a large bowl, combine parsnips, onion, seasonings and mix well.

Spoon mixture into a hot skillet and pat into skillet to flatten.

Cook over low heat about 15 to 20 minutes until tender and crisp. *Note: if you cook on high heat, the mixture will not cook, but rather will brown or burn.*

Cut with a spatula to make wedges and turn. Continue to cook about 5 more minutes or until the other side is golden and slightly crispy.

If sensitive to onion, you can substitute garlic or eliminate it all together. You can also add a bit of Romano cheese to the mixture, which helps bind ingredients and give it a nice Italian flavor. I am occasionally able to locate Romano-type cheese made from goats' milk.

❋ *Historical Matters—In the Middle Ages, especially during Lent, Europeans favored the parsnip because of its flavor, nourishment and ability to satisfy hunger through meatless fasting periods. In fact, parsnips once enjoyed greater popularity than either potatoes or carrots.*

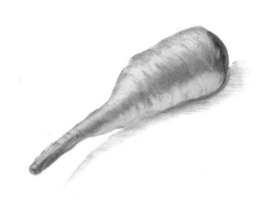

Gingered Sweet Potatoes

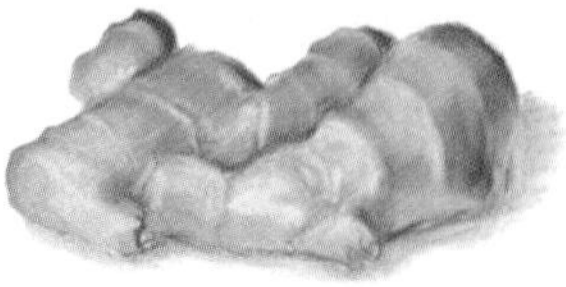

4 well-scrubbed, sweet potatoes
2 cloves crushed garlic
1 tsp Braggs™ Amino Acids
3 T organic butter or coconut oil (softened)
1/2 inch piece of fresh ginger, peeled and very finely chopped
1/2 cup sesame seeds

Prick the skins of the sweet potatoes with a sharp knife. Bake at 350°F for 1 hour or until tender when poked with a fork.

While the sweet potatoes are baking, combine the softened butter or coconut oil with chopped ginger and crushed garlic, and set aside.

Place the sesame seeds into a dry skillet and toss over very low heat for about 2 minutes until golden brown. Remove from skillet, place seeds between paper towels or a soft cloth and, with a rolling pin or blunt object, gently crush sesame seeds to release more of their aroma. Remove seeds from skillet and set aside.

After baking, and while still hot, cut the sweet potatoes into wedges and mix into it the softened butter or coconut oil with ginger and garlic and top with Braggs™ Amino Acids and roasted sesame seeds—serve warm. This dish can be baked ahead and simply reheated; it gets better when it's had time to absorb the mixture of flavors.

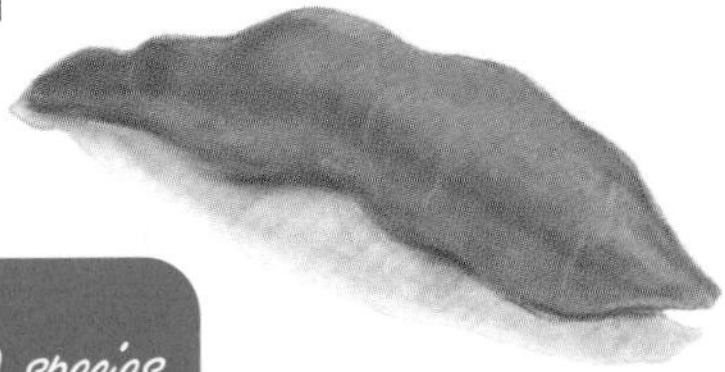

History of the Yam – There are over 150 species of yams grown in the world. Most yams sold in the U.S., however, are actually sweet potatoes. (Yams are higher in sugar than sweet potatoes.)

This thick, tropical-vine tuber is popular in South and Central America, the West Indies and parts of Asia and Africa. Although sweet potatoes and yams are similar in many ways and therefore often confused with one another, they are from different plant species.

Sweet Soufflé

1 1/2 cup baked, peeled, and mashed sweet potatoes
2 eggs
1/4 cup cream or milk substitute
1/2 cup honey or natural sweetener like SweetLife® to taste
1/4 tsp ginger powder
1 tsp cinnamon powder
1/4 tsp clove powder

Place mashed sweet potatoes in a bowl and beat with electric mixer as you slowly add all the remaining ingredients—blend until smooth.

Pour mixture in a buttered baking dish.
Bake at 375°F for 35 to 40 minutes.

Best when served warm, but also tasty cold as a side dish.

✳ *Can be served as a dessert topped with whipped cream or ice cream (rice dream).*

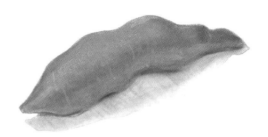

Dilly Partatos

4 chopped green onions
4 T butter or coconut oil
8-10 parsnips, peeled and sliced very thin
2 garlic cloves, finely minced
1 1/2 cup half & half or milk substitute
3/4 cup freshly grated soft goat cheese or other soft cheese
1 tsp dill weed

Sauté onion and garlic in butter or coconut oil. Add the remaining ingredients and heat over low heat until hot.

Pour the mixture into a greased casserole dish and bake at 350°F covered for 40 minutes. Remove cover and continue to bake for an additional 20 minutes.

N.F. (Nightshade-FREE) Vichyssoise

Trim tops off of leeks and thinly slice just the white portion of leeks, should measure about 1 cup.

In a saucepan, add leeks, onion, carrots and butter and sauté until tender *but not brown*.

Add sliced parsnips, chicken broth and salt to taste. Bring to gentle boil and reduce heat. Cover and simmer approx. 30 minutes until parsnips are extremely tender.

Let mixture cool but still warm. Place half the mixture into a blender or food processor and blend until velvety smooth. Pour blended mixture into a large bowl or large saucepan. Continue to blend the remainder of the mixture.

Return blended mixture in a saucepan and add milk or milk substitute. Bring to boil making sure to continue stirring to avoid burning and clumping.

Cool and stir in half and half or heavy cream. Cover and chill at least 2 hours, preferably overnight for best flavor.

Garnish with snipped chives

If using milk substitute, you may need to thicken the mixture. If so, place milk substitute in a measuring cup and add 2 to 3 T of rice or tapioca flour and blend well with whisk to avoid clumps. When mixture is smooth, you can slowly add as directed in recipe.

4 leeks
2 med. sized onions, sliced
2 T organic butter
3 cup parsnips, peeled and thinly sliced
2 cup half-and-half or heavy cream
1 1/2 cup milk or milk substitute (rice or goat milk)*
Snips of chives
2 cups low-salt chicken broth
2 med. carrots, peeled and grated on a fine grater

✳ *This cold soup is also great served with a dollop of sour cream or fresh made goat milk cream. . .it adds a rich sharp taste.*

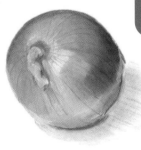

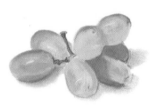

2 bunches green
seedless grapes, cut
lengthwise (canned
or frozen may be
used)
2 large beets (cooked,
peeled and sliced in
shoestrings)—you can
use more or less of
the above depending
on your taste
1/2 tsp powdered sugar
or SweetLife™ to
taste (adjust
sweetness to allow
for an overall
delicate sweetness
Juice of 1/4 fresh lemon
2 T mayonnaise

6 medium sweet
potatoes (scrubbed
and slightly pierced)

Green & Red Salad

*This is my favorite salad for the holidays or a hot
summer day (you won't even miss that potato
salad); it's colorful, low in calories, easy and is my
substitute for those occasions when you just want a
light, refreshing salad that's unique, of course.*

Place all the ingredients into a large mixing
bowl and mix well. Refrigerate overnight. Serve
chilled on lettuce leaves.

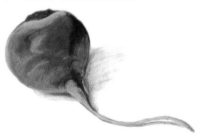

Oven-baked Taters

*Okay, I know these are not baked potatoes, I can tell
you, however, they're delicious. They have their own
naturally addictive taste and consistency, try them.*

Sweet potatoes should only be baked slow and
at low temperatures, about 300ºF. It's hard to
estimate how long cooking time will be—as soon
as the sweet potato feels slightly soft when
squeezed with an oven mitt, they're done. Usual
time is 60 to 90 minutes at 300ºF for medium-sized
potatoes.

Garnishing Options—Butter, sweet cream,
powdered cinnamon, or chives.

❋ *Storing Beets –
Loosely wrap in paper
towel and keep in
refrigerator crisper
for up to one week.
They can also be kept
in a root cellar or
other cool location.*

Fries, Home-Style

These are my favorites for breakfast or brunch with eggs and nightshade and nitrate-free bacon.

Melt butter or coconut in fry pan. If using coconut oil, be sure to slowly heat on medium heat, otherwise, you'll set off the smoke detectors—I've done it.

Add onion, potatoes and garlic and cook until brown and soft.

Note—Sometimes sweet potatoes are difficult to cook and take longer than conventional potatoes. If you'd like to speed the cooking process, precook the sweet potatoes a bit in the conventional oven and then proceed with directions above. I personally use a convection toaster oven with great success.

Options—You can replace the sweet potato with yucca root or parsnip, delicious seasoned with a dash of dill, cumin or coriander.

3 large sweet potatoes (scrubbed and sliced)
3 T butter or coconut oil
1 large onion (diced)
Salt (to taste)
2 cloves garlic (minced) optional

✻ *Dr. G's favorite: Jewel sweet potato, try several varieties to identify your favorite*

Italian Garlic Roasted Parsnips

I love garlic. This recipe is down-right satisfying. It transforms the humble, under-rated parsnip into a side-dish rave of crispy brown decadence.

In a small saucepan over low heat, cook the oil and garlic until garlic is pale beige (do not brown). Remove from heat, add the rosemary, cover and steep for 30 minutes.

Preheat oven to 400°F. Strain the oil into a roasting pan large enough to hold the parsnips in one layer.

In the original saucepan or large bowl, add parsnips, salt, and pepper and toss to completely cover ingredients.

Bake in the top of the oven. Turn parsnips occasionally with tongs until they are crispy and tender (approx. 40 minutes). Sprinkle the balsamic vinegar and toss; take another 5 to 10 minutes. Serve immediately.

1/2 cup extra virgin oil
5 garlic cloves, (minced or crushed)
3 three-inch springs fresh rosemary or 2 tsp dried rosemary
2 1/2 lbs parsnips (peeled and cut into one inch chunks)
1 tsp salt
1/2 tsp fresh ground pepper
2 T balsamic vinegar

51

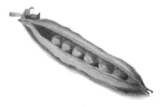

Balkan Parsnip & Pea Salad

*A staple of many western European countries, this side dish has a hardy, deep, and heart-warming flavor. Serve **hot** as a side dish or **cold** as a great picnic salad (see below).*

2 lbs. *unpeeled* parsnips (well-scrubbed)
3 stalks celery (cut into 1/8 inch slices)
1 1/2 cup thawed or fresh baby peas
1/4 tsp salt
1/4 tsp fresh ground white pepper
1/4 tsp fresh basil leaves (coarsely chopped) for garnish
1 yellow onion (coarsely chopped) *for hot side dish only

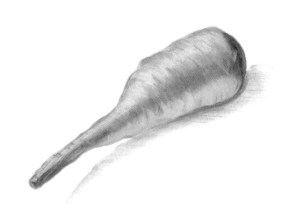

1/2 cup fresh Parmesan cheese
1/4 cup firmly-packed fresh basil leaves (coarsely chopped)
3 T balsamic vinegar
1 T red wine vinegar
1/2 tsp salt
1/4 tsp fresh ground black pepper
3/4 cup extra-virgin olive oil

BALKAN PESTO VINAIGRETTE

Make vinaigrette by combining all ingredients, excluding the oil, in a blender. While the blender is still running, gradually add the oil until the dressing is smooth and silky.

Options—serve **cold** or **hot** (see below):

COLD SALAD—Bring a large pot of salted water to a boil over high heat. Add the parsnips and cook, uncovered, until they're tender (not soft) when pierced with a knife (approx. 20 minutes). Drain and rinse under cold water. After cooling, slice into 1/2 inch thick rounds and place in a large bowl.

Add the celery, peas, and 3/4 of the dressing. Cover and refrigerate for at least 4 hours, best if overnight. Toss with the remaining dressing, salt, and pepper.

Garnish with basil leaves and serve chilled.

HOT SIDE-DISH—Follow directions above for cooking parsnips except remove from water when consistency is al dente (cooked but firm). After cooling and slicing set aside. In a large sauté pan or skillet, warm butter or a small amount of oil enough to sauté onions and celery. Cook onions until lightly brown. Add cooked/sliced parsnips and peas and continue cooking until soft but not overcooked. Add vinaigrette until warmed and serve. For the best blend of flavors, make ahead several hours or the day before serving, and reheat.

Word *Matters*

AL DENTE is a fancy term for pasta or vegetables that are fully cooked, but not overly soft. The phrase is Italian for "to the tooth," which comes from testing the pasta's consistency with the teeth.

Derived from the Italian words: al (to the) + dente (tooth)

❋ *The food value of parsnips exceeds that of any other vegetable except potatoes. They are easily grown, therefore should be farmed more extensively.*

Caramelized Parsnip Frittata

1 lb. parsnips (unpeeled and well-scrubbed)
2 T olive oil
1 tsp salt
1/4 tsp fresh ground pepper
10 large eggs
3 tsp fresh rosemary (chopped) or 1 tsp. dried rosemary
3 oz extra-sharp raw cheddar cheese or goat cheese

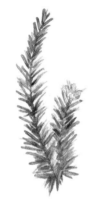

3 T unsalted butter or coconut oil
3 large yellow onions (cut into 1/8 inch thick half moons)
1/4 tsp salt
1/8 tsp freshly ground black pepper
3 T balsamic vinegar
1 1/2 tsp sugar

This dish will get you rave reviews whether served for brunch, lunch, or dinner. Served with a hearty salad, it becomes a healthy, complete meatless meal.

Cook parsnips in salted water over high heat for 10 minutes, until par-boiled. Drain and rinse under cold water until cooled enough to cut into 1/2 inch thick slices.

In a 10-inch oven-proof non-stick skillet, heat the oil over medium heat. Add the parsnips, salt and pepper. Be sure to arrange in skillet as evenly as possible. Cook, uncovered, turning the parsnips occasionally until browned and tender for approx. 15 minutes.

Prepare the broiler rack about 6 inches from the heat elements and preheat.

In a large bowl, whisk the eggs, rosemary, salt and pepper until well mixed. Pour over the parsnips and reduce heat to medium-low. Lift the cooked part of the frittata to allow the egg mixture to flow underneath. Continue cooking until the top is set. Sprinkle top with cheese of choice. Broil until the frittata is puffed, browned and set. Before serving, spread the warm caramelized onions on top.

CARAMELIZED ONION TOPPING

In a medium nonstick skillet, melt the butter or oil over medium heat. Add the sliced onions, salt and pepper. Cook, stirring often to avoid scorching, until onions are soft and deep golden brown. Stir in the balsamic vinegar and sugar and cook until the vinegar is reduced to a glaze. Keep the mixture warm to pour over frittata. This mixture can be made, and is actually tastier, up to two days in advance when kept covered and refrigerated.

Vegetable Strudel

A light, crispy, satisfying main course when accompanied by a salad and also a great replacement for a starch. You can stuff with any vegetable.

Unroll filo dough, using two sheets at a time. Cover the remaining dough with a damp towel to keep moist. Brush filo with melted butter, adding the second sheet and brushing it with melted butter. Be sure to work quickly so dough does not dry out.

Prepare all other ingredients as directed and mix in a large bowl.

Add 1/2 of the filling and roll into a rectangular piece, like a burrito, folding in side edges. Repeat the procedure until all the filling is used.

Place on greased baking sheet or use parchment paper. Brush with butter and bake at 400°F for 15 to 20 minutes until medium golden brown. Serve warm.

4 sheets filo dough (thawed)
1/2 cup butter (melted)
1 cup spinach (steamed & chopped)
1/2 cup ricotta cheese
1 egg (beaten)
1/2 cup zucchini (sliced thin & sautéed)
1 cup marinated artichoke hearts (oil drained)
1 cup mushrooms (sliced & sautéed)
1/2 sweet potato (roasted, cooled, peeled & sliced thin)
3 T basil (fresh)
1/2 cup pine nuts (gently roasted in cast iron skillet & chopped)

Historical *Matters*

BALSAMIC VINEGAR—The Italians call it *aceto balsamico tradizionale*, a delicacy rarely known outside of Italy until twenty-five years ago—mostly made and used by wealthy families in small towns for over a thousand years who passed it on as a family heirloom, given to esteemed friends in small vials, or bequeathed to a daughter as part of her dowry. Although thought to be made from *wine, it is not.* It is made from the *un*fermented juice from grapes. These sweet grapes are then pressed and the pressings are cooked-down to a dark syrup (a reduction sauce). The syrup is then placed into small oak barrels containing a vinegar "mother" left from previous years. This starts the aging process. It is used medicinally for everything from warding off evil spirits to stimulating the appetite, restoring tranquility, curing colds, treating heart conditions, preventing insomnia and soothing throat inflammations.

Avoid cayenne, chili powder, ground red pepper, crushed red pepper, curry, and paprika.

INSTEAD OF TOMATOES

Whatever you use tomatoes for the alternatives are only limited by your willingness to be healthy and creative. Whether it be salad dressings, pasta sauces, pizza topping, your favorite roast, or that mouth-watering B.B.Q. sauce, hopefully these healthy alternatives will "plant the seed" of creativity for you to create tasty meals without the pain and inflammation from nightshades.

Salsa, My Way

1 cup chopped fresh pineapple
Other substitutes for pineapple include: papaya, mango or kiwi
(increase lime juice to add acidity).
1 cup chopped fresh cantaloupe, honeydew or water melon
1/2 cup finely chopped strawberries or red currents
2 finely chopped oranges or pink grapefruit, seeded
6 finely chopped green onions or scallions
1/2 cup finely chopped fresh cilantro
The juice of 1 to 2 limes

There's absolutely no reason to give up that delicious salsa as a dip with your favorite tacos, or ethnic meal. When I first served this sweet version to my guests, I could only image what they were thinking "Okay, this time she's definitely gone over the edge, I can't even imagine sweet salsa on my chicken tacos". By the middle of the meal everyone was having two and three helpings of salsa, and by the end of the meal there was no salsa left...before everyone went home they wanted the recipe. This recipe is limited only by your imagination; try it as a pizza topping too, it's delicious.

Mix all ingredients together and add lime juice; refrigerate 2 hours before serving. Adjust fruit as needed for your particular dietary needs and availability.

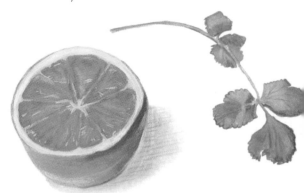

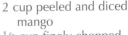
Tequila Sunrise Salsa

This salsa is exceptional but does contain liquor. I find that in small amounts used for culinary purposes, even sensitive digestive systems do not react negatively. If you're sensitive to alcohol, try apple cider vinegar, sake, or non-alcoholic white wine.

Combine ingredients in a small bowl and stir well. Cover and chill at least 2 hours. Makes about 2 cups.

Great used as a marinade and/or sauce for fish and chicken.

2 cup peeled and diced mango
1/2 cup finely chopped celery
3 T tequila
2 T orange juice
2 tsp finely chopped fresh mint
Salt & pepper to taste

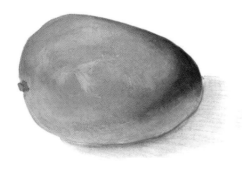

Tomato *Matters*

Beware of: ketchup, spaghetti sauce, tomato juice, bloody Mary mix, V-8 juice, sun-dried tomatoes and pizza. Avoid steak sauces, Worcestershire, Tabasco, barbecue, and brown sauces that contain nightshades in the form of peppers and spices.

❋ *Pumpkin and seasonings make an excellent substitute for duplicating the taste and texture of tomatoes.*

Plum-Good BBQ Sauce, My Way

8 plums, pitted and chopped fine (may use sour cherries or a combination)

1 T oil

1 medium onion, minced extremely fine

1/4 cup apple cider vinegar (can use red wine vinegar)

The juice of one lemon

4 T Mt. Capra Mineral Whey powder (or brown sugar)

1 1/2 tsp dry mustard

Salt and pepper to taste

1/4 tsp ground cloves

4 cloves garlic, minced extremely fine

1/2 cup pureed cooked beets with juice

This sauce is amazing; a true example of the old saying "necessity is the mother of invention." Remember to adjust the ingredients according to your taste buds, I like a true, sharp taste, you may not.

Sauté onion and garlic over medium heat until tender but not brown.

Mix all ingredients with electric or hand mixer, in a bowl until well blended.

Return mixture to saucepan and slowly cook for 1 hour, taking caution to stir frequently so it doesn't burn or stick.

Taste and adjust flavor to your satisfaction, you may want to add more mineral whey for added sweetness, or add more liquid with additional beet juice, or even add more plums.

Best flavor is accomplished when refrigerated at least overnight. It also freezes well, so once you get the recipe the way you like it, you can double the quantity and freeze.

• *Use this as a marinade or before grilling burgers, steaks or chicken.*

• *If sauce is too thin, thicken with a bit of rice flour dissolved in beet juice and cook an additional 20 minutes to desired consistency.*

• *You can also add hickory flavored liquid smoke but be sure it's nightshade-free*

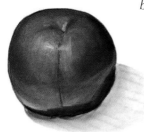

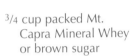

Sweet & Sour Sauce

Dissolve mineral whey and rice flour in warmed pineapple juice.

In a small saucepan, combine the above mixture and stir in the remaining ingredients.

Cook over medium-high heat, stirring constantly until thickened and bubbly. Continue to cook 3 to 5 minutes until garlic is soft. May serve warm as a topper for spareribs or Asian dishes.

3/4 cup packed Mt. Capra Mineral Whey or brown sugar

1 T rice flour

1/3 cup red wine vinegar

1/3 cup unsweetened pineapple juice (may use finely chopped pineapple and juice)

1 T Braggs™ Amino Acids or low sodium soy sauce

1 garlic clove, minced extremely fine

1/4 tsp ground ginger

2 kiwi, peeled and chopped fine (optional)

1/2 tsp dry mustard (adjust to your taste)

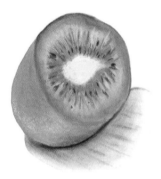

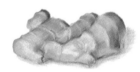

Deli *Matters*

Avoid baked beans, bologna, deli meats, frankfurters, meat loaf, turkey bacon, pastrami, corned beef, sausage, and many salad dressings as they contain hidden nightshades like paprika and cayenne.

Cranberry BBQ Sauce

2-12 oz. bags fresh
cranberries (minced)
(if using dried berries
be sure to soak)
1 Maui onion
(finely minced)
2 garlic cloves
(finely minced)
1/2 to 2/3 cup Capra
Mineral Whey™ or
brown sugar
1/2 cup apple cider
vinegar
1/4 cup balsamic
vinegar
1/2 cup crystallized
orange peel
(finely minced)
1 fresh lime
(peeled & minced)
1 fresh lemon
(peeled & minced)
1 small can frozen
orange juice (pure,
unsweetened)
1 tsp grated fresh ginger
1/3 cup honey
1/4 tsp meat tenderizer*
Salt & pepper to taste

*Use any full-spectrum
digestive enzyme
powder or open
capsules.

An exotic, tenderizing marinade great for any meat except ground. It's not too sweet with a zest that keeps beckoning an Asian influence. Whoever said we'd miss conventional tomato-based BBQ sauces isn't very adventurous.

Place cranberries in pan with 1/2 cup water and cook slowly for about 15 minutes.

Sauté onion and garlic in 1 T oil until soft then add to cranberries and mix with the remainder of uncooked ingredients.

Mix ingredients well and coat chicken, ribs, turkey, steaks overnight or at least 2 hrs.

This is a thick, rich sauce that replaces traditional tomato base.

Ribs—Cook in boiling water for about 20 minutes. Cool then marinade as described above.

Roasts—You might want to marinade overnight, then sprinkle with rice flour and brown in coconut oil before roasting.

Chicken, Cornish Hens and Turkey—It is advisable to inject the bird if possible with a meat injector to get the flavor from the inside out. Marinade only 1 hour and use 1/8 tsp. of tenderizer per bird. If you do not own a meat injector, it will be one of the best investments you can make. However, you can also purchase a veterinarian broad-tipped needle and do the same. Make sure if injecting that you blend the ingredients so it will not jam the injector.

Ground meat—Not advisable to use the tenderizer because it makes the meat sticky. Use the recipe and omit the tenderizer.

Nutty Pesto Sauce

This sauce is so versatile you'll want to make an extra jar. It's delicious served over your favorite pasta, grilled chicken or fish, or a delightful addition to any sandwich, especially tuna. Try tossing it into a green salad with your favorite vinaigrette, it's delicate and fragrant.

Roast pine nuts in dry heavy bottom pan until light tan (best if cast iron skillet).

Sauté shallots in 1 T of oil, just until soft.

Add everything into blender and mix well.

May refrigerate in glass jar for up to 1 week.

Adjust cilantro or basil to your taste. I've put as much as $1/2$ c. of chopped cilantro.

1 cup olive oil
2 cups fresh cilantro (coarsely chopped)
$1/3$ cup fresh chives or green onions (coarsely chopped)
2 shallots (peeled, chopped)*
$1/2$ cup pine nuts (roasted)
$1/4$ cup packed fresh mint leaves
1 glove fresh garlic
3 T of fresh lime juice
Salt & pepper to taste

*optional

East Meets West Vinaigrette Dressing

A fragrant, delicate dressing that can be mixed into a salad, used as a topping for pasta, or as a sandwich spread.

Place whole coriander seeds in a dry heavy bottom skillet on medium heat. Toast until a nice aroma (about 4 minutes). Cool and grind in mortar and pestle or spice mill.

Heat 1 T of oil in the same skillet, add shallots and sauté until soft but not brown, set aside and cool.

Mix all the ingredients in a bowl, mix well and refrigerate. Can be kept in a tightly sealed jar for about one week.

1 T coriander seeds (toasted)
$1/2$ cup olive oil
$1/4$ cup shallots (minced)
1 T balsamic vinegar
1 T apple cider vinegar
1 clove garlic (minced)
Salt

Parisian Balsamic Vinaigrette

½ cup balsamic
  vinegar
2 T olive Oil
2 T brewers Yeast
Salt and pepper to taste
4 cloves garlic (peeled
  and cut)

This is a dense, thick dressing that imparts that special flavor found in Parisian Bistros. It thickens as it sets, so it should be made the night before serving. Use as an exotic salad dressing or marinade for chicken or fish.

Mix all ingredients in a blender and blend until smooth. Place in a jar and refrigerate overnight for best flavor. Adjust oil for desired thickness.

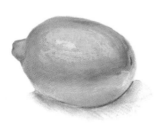

Lemon Basil Pesto Sauce

½ cup olive oil
¼ cup black olives
  (finely chopped)
½ tsp dill weed
  (crushed in mortar
  or spice mill)
½ fresh lemon (juiced)
½ cup fresh basil
  (finely chopped)
2 T rice vinegar
1 clove garlic (optional)

A delicious light sauce tossed with angel hair pasta, or served over chicken or fish.

Heat the oil and sauté all ingredients until tender and bubbly about 4-5 minutes. It is best if made in advance at least one hour before serving (preferably overnight) and reheated prior to serving.

You may also brown a chicken breast then pour this sauce over it and continue to slowly cook until tender; you may also do the same with fish. I've breaded my fish with a light rice flour mix, or Panco™ breading, browned and topped with warmed sauce.

HINTS—Many recipes call for stock or broth made from chicken, beef, or vegetables. The best choice is to make it homemade, that way you can rest assured it does not contain nightshades.

After cooking your favorite stock, cool then refrigerate to allow fat to coagulate for easy removal. Place defatted soup into ice cube trays and freeze. Remove from trays and place in air-tight containers for easy use. This is a great, convenient way to always be prepared with homemade broth or stock.

You may do the same with a reduction stock, which is much tastier thick, rich, and concentrated.

Tarragon Alfredo Sauce

This is about as rich as a sauce gets! Use it over fettuccini noodles, or as a dense sauce for chicken.

Heat butter until melted and lightly brown the flour until a light golden clump forms, not brown. Slowly add half-and-half or milk, salt and pepper to taste, *stirring continually to avoid lumps.* Cook over medium heat until thickness desired. Add the wine and fresh tarragon, cook approx. 1 minute and serve.

Note—You may thicken or thin sauce by increasing or decreasing liquid and flour until desired consistency.

Options—

•Add plain yogurt or sour cream for a velvety sauce.

•Add 1 T sherry after removing from heat, instead of wine.

•Substitute for any recipe that calls for canned celery or cream of chicken soup. To achieve the desired flavor, add celery, mushrooms, chicken broth etc.

2 cups traditional
   white sauce roux*
1/4 cup white wine (may
   use non-alcoholic
   wine or sake)
2 T fresh tarragon
   (finely minced)

* Dr. G's white
  sauce roux:
3 cups half-and-half
   (milk substitute,
   or milk)
1/2 cup rice flour
   (may use wheat
   or tapioca flour)
4-6 T butter

Mexican Red Sauce

Mix ingredients together in a bowl and refrigerate at least 1 hour before serving.

Options—

•For more "fire" add additional horseradish or white pepper and a bit more apple cider vinegar.

•This sauce freezes well for future use.

1 1lb. can pumpkin
   (Libby brand has no
   food-coloring)
1/2 tsp salt
1 onion (finely minced)
3/4 tsp coriander
1 T horseradish
1/2 cup water
1/4 cup apple cider vinegar
2 cloves garlic (finely minced)
1 T cumin
1/2 T oregano (ground)
Black pepper (to taste)
Pinch of sugar or SweetLife®
   natural sweetener

❊ Dr. G's Favorite: I like this sauce for Mexican dishes like enchiladas and casseroles.

Dr. G's Guacamole

No recipe section would be complete without a guacamole recipe that didn't contain tomatoes. Try this on salads, tostadas, tacos, pizzas, quesadillas, grilled cheese sandwiches, chip-n-dip, and roll-ups.

4 lg. avocado (ripened)
3 T fresh lime juice
1/2 small red onion (diced)
2 garlic cloves (minced)
4 T fresh cilantro (minced)
3 T ranch dressing (nightshade-free) May increase to taste and desired consistency or substitute mayonnaise, or plain yogurt

Halve the avocados and remove the pits. Scoop out and mash until velvety smooth.

Squeeze lime juice into mixture and add remaining ingredients.

Add salt to taste and mix well.

Chill at least 2 hrs. before serving; lime juice prevents turning dark.

Enjoy, bon appetite.

Optional—Add a bit of crumbled goat-cheese or finely grated sharp jack or cheddar.

Dr. G's Teriyaki & Marinade Sauce

2 cup soy sauce (nightshade-free) or Bragg's Amino Acids™
2 T Saki (Japanese rice wine)
1/4 to 1/3 cup pineapple juice
3/4 cup brown or raw sugar (may use SweetLife™ natural sweetener, to taste)
4 T cornstarch, tapioca or rice flour (for thickening)
8 T cold water

In a saucepan over medium heat mix all ingredients except thickening agent used and water.

In a mixing cup with pouring spout, dissolve thickening agent in water. Slowly add to the soy sauce mixture when it's near boiling. Stir constantly until mixture reaches a consistency of thick and dark. Remove from heat.

Note—

•Everyone likes varied flavors from soy sauce and sugar, adjust to your taste.

•Marinating: Keep in mind that marinating enhances flavor and tenderizes. If using as a marinade, my preference is to marinade overnight, or at least two hours.

Dr. G's "Healthy Start" Shake

Dozens of clients, readers, and my radio listening audience, contact my office asking for the recipe for my protein shake that I have every morning and use while traveling. What you asked for Matters, here it is:

Place in blender with 8 to 10 oz of water.

For traveling—I pre-measure all the dry ingredients into small plastic snack bags and mix with a battery-operated blender. It provides me quick, sustained energy no matter where I go....especially when I find myself "stuck" in an airport since I don't eat fast food.

Options—You may add fruit, assuming you don't have a candida-yeast problem or blood sugar considerations. I especially like it with fresh cherries, strawberries, papaya or mango.

- 2 T Goatein™ (natural goat-milk protein powder without the fat)
- 2 T SweetWheat™ (organic, kosher, freeze-dried wheat grass juice powder—does not contain gluten)
- 2 T CapraFlex™ (a proprietary blend of botanicals, whole-food compounds, enzymes, and minerals providing powerful support for healthy joints, pain and inflammation)
- 2 T Udo's brand™ Oil blend (must refrigerate)
- 1 packet SweetLife™ Natural Sweetener (made from Lo Han)
- 2 T Capra Mineral Whey™ (pre-digested, mineral/electrolyte replacement made from natural goat-milk whey)

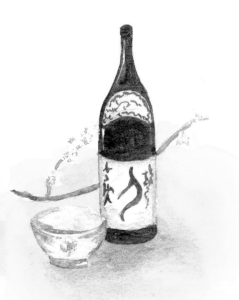

Section 4
Non-drug Pain & Inflammation Phyters

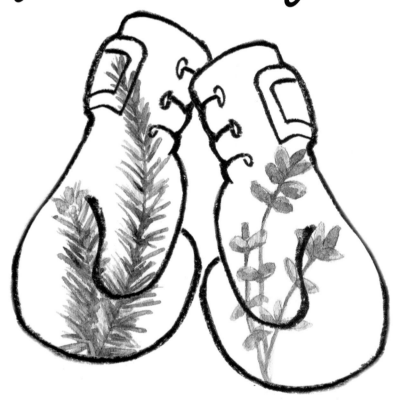

A Biological Approach to Healthy Joints, Pain & Inflammation

DEFINING BIOLOGICAL MEDICINE

First of all, since the basis for this book deals with biological medicine, allow me to define it. This newer term for non-drug methodologies simply means getting to the cause of the disorder or discomfort, not merely treating "symptoms" for a short-term "fix," serving only to mask or suppress underlying causes. The definition of biological medicine has best been summarized by Dr. Paavo Airola as metabolic disorders and chemical imbalances in the organs, glands, bones, and tissues of the body.

Pain & Inflammation Matter

Pain and Inflammation, without an actual injury such as a fracture, strain or sprain, is our body's way of attempting to deal with toxic overload. Many illnesses, and nearly all injuries, result in inflammatory reactions to a certain degree. However, in the absence of an injury, pain and inflammation are symptoms with some common denominators: leaky gut syndrome, toxic colon, over/burdened liver and lymph system, consumption of nightshade foods, and the resulting immune system dysfunction. This is evident in related conditions such as fibromyalgia, chronic fatigue, myofascial pain syndrome, lupus, arthritis, psoriasis, and scleroderma to mention a few.

Today, we have the opportunity to avoid prescription drugs, except for short-term use in acute cases, and use natural substances, dietary changes and environmental modifications that not only effectively give symptom-relief, but also assist in reversing causes of the discomfort.

Definition Matters

According to Merriam-Webster, tenth edition, biological pertains to "life and living processes."

Pain and inflammation is also *not* unique to the 10 million people in the U.S. currently diagnosed with **Osteoporosis**, and the additional 24 million who have been identified as having a low bone-mass index. **Pain and inflammation** are also daily companions for the estimated 26 million suffering from the group of disorders previously mentioned.

pH & Bone Health Matter

Research confirms that the standard American diet, high in meat and low in alkalizing fruits and vegetables, leaves an acid residue in the body; associated with bone loss and low bone density. The only minerals I found that perform the job of supporting bone health, muscle integrity *and* neutralizing acid waste better than any other form are minerals derived from fresh, free-ranged, goat-milk whey. It's an innovative concept, but not a new one.

In addition to containing more than twenty naturally-occurring minerals necessary for peak performance, goat-milk whey contains healthy amounts of sodium to control acid-alkaline balances, essential for healthy muscles and bones. This type of goat-milk whey has been used for decades to promote bone density as well as for its ability to relieve aching, painful joints and connective tissue pain as that in fibromyalgia sufferers.

> ✳ With over 70 million baby boomers joining the 50-plus group, including this author, the need to educate ourselves in non-drug options for prevention, control and reversal of these disorders is now more crucial than ever.

Golden Matters

It is said that in parts of Eastern Europe, goat-milk whey is sold for more money per ounce than gold.

Salt: A Habit Worth Shaking

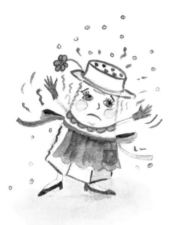

Recently, there have been a surge of new products that claim to be healthy salt alternatives or substitutes—*buyer beware*. Many of these alternatives still contain sodium chloride, the same substance contained in regular salt.

Additionally, consumers have been advised that "natural" salt is healthier; Yes, it is in a healthy individual without a condition of hypertension or inflammation. However, that said, salt in any form still has the propensity to elevate blood pressure and increase fluid retention in tissues, causing inflammation and pain.

The naturally-occurring sodium contained in a whole food such as mineral whey should not be confused with salt, they are not the same.

NECESSITY IS THE MOTHER OF INVENTION

Okay, I'm a gourmet cook and you hate to cook, or you're in poor health and cooking is the last thing you need to add to your "must do" list. However, if you're going to "shake" the salt habit and replace it with tasty, healthy alternatives you must get creative.

Decide what herbs and spices have flavors you enjoy and to which you are not sensitive. Then make your own special seasonings—soon you won't miss the salt, and you've still enhanced everything you eat. Don't be surprised if family and friends start asking for the recipe, mine did.

Try a combination of herbs/seasonings and name them something exotic that becomes your own blend. Just remember to write exact ingredients and amounts so when it's a "winner" you can reproduce it—speaking from experience, *naturally.* Ingredients that make a good seasoning blend include:

- dried onion and garlic (be sure to make it yourself or buy organic, nightshade-free)
- thyme
- rosemary
- cumin
- coriander
- marjoram
- celery seed
- dried lemon powder (buy pure, beware of additives)
- oregano
- citrus peel
- mustard
- cilantro
- basil
- black, pink, and while peppercorns

Remember: Salt intake MUST be controlled in order to combat inflammation and other known health effects of salt intake such as hypertension.

Solutions for Fibromyalgia (FM)

FIBROMYALGIA: LOSS OF HORMONE FITNESS

According to many nutritional experts, Fibromyalgia is attributed to loss of hormone fitness. This lost fitness is due to the hypothalamus gland literally being exhausted, not able to effectively carry out its work of ensuring hormones are kept in natural balance.

A condition called Leptin resistance, and related issues, actually set the stage for hormone exhaustion. The hormones are still in the blood; however, they can no longer do the work the way they did when we were hormonally fit (in balance).

Salt Matters

It was enlightening to me while researching for the past few years, for both this book and to continue to improve my health, that I had been using so much salt. Years ago I only used a minimal amount in my cooking. After recovering from my chemical sensitivities and subsequent digestive disorders, I craved more and more salt...until it became evident it was a large part of my on-again, off-again soft tissue symptoms. As soon as I restricted salt intake, I felt the overall improvement/ elimination of fluid retention, muscle stress and tissue inflammation.

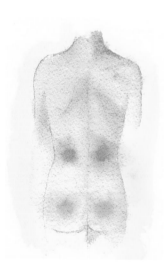

The solution is to do everything possible to stop fibromyalgia hormone imbalance in the first place by some of the measures mentioned elsewhere in this book and supplementation with Lipoic acid, to alleviate pain and nerve inflammation.

- *Lipoic acid*—A potent antioxidant for the damage associated from the excess production of NF kappaB. Numerous studies demonstrate the ability of lipoic acid to turn off the production of excess NF kappaB which occurs as the proteins of muscle fiber are cemented together in abnormal structures and cause pain. The longer a person stays in the fibromyalgia pain condition, the more likely damage is being done to the muscles; lipoic acid helps stop the progression of tissue damage. The most effective form of lipoic acid is called R alpha lipoic acid.

Other nutrients that also assist in repairing tissue damage and inflammation, which contribute to the overall hormone imbalance, are bromelain, papain, DL phenylalanine, boswellia and curcumin (*see section on Additional Phyters*). These nutrients help to dissolve the abnormal tissue protein and reduce the tissue toxic load that contributes to imbalances in general.

New Views on Fibromyalgia
Reduction of Stored Toxins: Effective for Pain, Inflammation and Weight Loss

In order to reduce toxins stored in the soft and connective tissues, the individual must get the intestinal plumbing to flow (detoxification of the large intestine). The toxins in the blood, as well as stored toxins that come out of fat cells when weight is lost must have some place to go. The body is reluctant to break down toxic fat if there is no place to send the toxins—the old cliché of creating a void before it can again fill. That said, when the intestinal plumbing is clogged or sluggish, the body seeks a secondary storage for toxic waste, that storage being fat cells and the lymphatic system; at least getting the toxic substances out of circulation and away from vital organs. The fibromyalgia patient experiences that "bruised all over feeling" as the soft and connective tissues shelter accumulated wastes.

In addition to getting intestinal plumbing to flow, fibromyalgia patients have difficulty losing weight because they do not release growth hormone (GH) in response to exercise, as healthy individuals do. Scientists surmise that the GH regulatory system no longer heeds its "signal" to keep the production factory working; in other words, it's tired from being subjected to prolonged stress and goes on strike until the overall metabolic stress is reduced.

To locate a retailer of the intestinal fiber cleanse tablets, CapraCleanse™, and EZGo™, the natural, non-habit-forming herbal stool softener used and recommended by Dr. G, see resource section.

The complete protocol for intestinal cleansing is discussed in the book *Invisible Illnesses*, available through this book's *Resource Section*, major booksellers and at www.drgloriagilbere.com.

Non-drug Pain & Inflammation Phyters

There are many "safe" options conventionally overlooked in the search for non-drug solutions. The following are, in my personal and professional experience, some of the most effective.

Experience *Matters*

It is imperative that intestinal cleansing and maintenance be performed before any protocol for pain and inflammation is successful. This volume, however, does not have space to provide those protocols in detail. Keep in mind; you MUST reduce the overall toxic load of the body before reversal of symptoms can be achieved.

Inflammation *Matters*

A review from the University of Washington, in Seattle, noted that vitamin E is a "chain-breaking" antioxidant with therapeutic potential to regulate inflammatory response by preventing intracellular signaling cascades within the inflammatory cells."

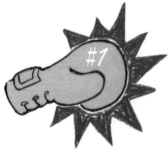

PHYTER #1: LIFESTYLE CHANGES

Challenge: It is common knowledge that although bone and joint pain is oftentimes caused by injury, it is also caused by arthritic degeneration (rheumatoid arthritis) of the joint itself. Yet nearly 21 million Americans suffer from the most common form of arthritis—osteoarthritis. In years past, it was believed osteoarthritis was simply caused by joints wearing, as in the aging process—yes, aging wear and tear are contributors. However, recent research show other variables are also contributing factors, including genetic predisposition and a disorder caused by an increase in enzymes that breakdown protoglycans and collagen. Symptoms of osteo-arthritis include:

- Joint pain and stiffness
- Joint swelling
- Stiffness made worse by inactivity
- Creaking joints
- Inflammation in soft and connective tissues
- Joint abnormalities

Another form of arthritis, fibromyalgia, is believed by some, including myself, to be caused by an over-burdened liver that can no longer protect us because of intestinal toxic overload.

Considerations: The phyte for prevention of osteoarthritis begins by protecting against injuries—insurance companies report that most accidents happen in the home or office. After an accident or trauma, the rate of arthritis related disorders, including fibromyalgia, increases by approximately 80%. The following are daily precautions to consider:

- Make sure your workplace has ergonomic accommodations for what are known as neutral body mechanics.
- Wear correct-fitting shoes—slip-ons can cause a slip-off and strain tendons/ligaments in knees, legs and calves.

- Be aware, practice good posture.
- Wear protective sports gear.
- Warm-up before workouts and don't overdue.
- Wear shoes that provide a grip for wet and icy weather, or use removable Ice Grippers.
- If your job requires hours of sitting, do some light stretching exercises like Pilates™ or Yoga to reduce stress and improve circulation.
- Wear a variety of shoe styles and varied heel heights to balance the wear on feet, legs, knees and hips.
- Never use a ladder that is not stable and preferably only use a high one when another person is in close proximity.

Goal: Reduce pain and inflammation, whether from an injury, wear-and-tear, or toxic overload.

Solution: Avoid all foods in the nightshade group and those that contain a poisonous substance called solanine, known to accelerate inflammation; tomatoes, potatoes, peppers (all varieties), eggplant, pimento, paprika, artichokes, huckleberries, and blueberries. Tobacco is also a nightshade; therefore smoking will accelerate an inflammatory condition (*see Nightshade-free Recipes, Section 3*). In addition, the following detoxification and lifestyle changes are imperative if you are to truly avoid and reverse pain and inflammation:

- Engage in a detoxification program for the colon, liver, kidneys and lymphatic system.
- Drink plenty of pure water (half of body weight in ounces).
- Avoid caffeine or limit intake to one cup per day.
- Maintain a healthy weight—overweight people are more likely to develop arthritis and wear out weight-bearing joints such as hips, knees and ankles.

UNDERSTANDING THE
JARGON—Bone, Joint,
Ligament, and Tendon
Health 101
• Glucosamine—What IT IS
and What IT DOES
  Glucosamine is
chondroprotective: an agent
that restores cartilage by
providing the material
needed for chondrocytes to
regenerate cartilage tissue. It

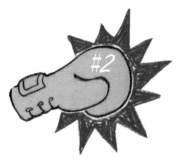

makes up the building blocks
in the body that build
cartilage, ease pain and
connective tissue
inflammation (as in
fibromyalgia and arthritis)
and acts as a general natural
anti-inflammatory.
  Glucosamine molecules are
quite small, allowing for rapid
absorption into the intestinal
tract, subsequently easily
distributed to bones and
cartilage. Because of rapid
absorption, sources of
glucosamine extracted from
crab, lobster or shrimp shells
are not considered a good
source because of the

continued on the next page

- Do regular dry-skin brushing to stimulate lymph flow.
- Exercise—it strengthens and cushions joints by releasing synovial fluid. If exercise is painful, walk, walk, walk at least five days per week for thirty minutes. The best combination is to start slow and rotate your exercise with stretching, aerobics and endurance training.
- Avoid excessive consumption of alcohol.
- Avoid excessive stress when possible.

PHYTER #2: BONE, LIGAMENT, TENDON, SOFT & CONNECTIVE TISSUE SUPPORT

Challenge: Disorders like fibromyalgia, which mostly affect the soft tissues, are not as easy to define with a set of symptoms or treat with a set of solutions. However, a doctor from Canada, Dr. Hugh Smythe, coined a phrase I feel most appropriate in describing its symptoms "The irritable everything syndrome." In fibromyalgia victims, there is not one particular type of cell or part of the body affected—the only commonality is that no two cases or symptoms are exactly the same. The one common denominator is that accumulated toxins are being redistributed and usually set-up house in the eighteen trigger points used to diagnose the disorder.

Goal: The goal in providing long-term reversal of fibromyalgia, and effectively combat bone and joint problems, is to first detoxify the body, specifically intestinal cleansing.

  The second is to provide as much natural support to the bones, ligaments, tendons and connective tissue while providing substances that will reduce pain and inflammation—not an easy task for a non-pharmaceutical product.

A Unique Solution

CapraFlex™, complete, comprehensive bone and joint health support formula, contains Type II chicken collagen, cartilage and bone-building compounds, providing the body what it needs to increase bone density while also rebuilding healthy cartilage and connective tissue.

Even more unique in this formula are whole foods, herbs and enzymes for pain associated with inflammation, especially helpful for soft tissue pain in fibromyalgia sufferers.

Why does Capraflex contain Type II Chicken Collagen?

Because Type II collagen (also known as CCII) is the principle structural protein in cartilage— providing strength, flexibility and joint support.

The CCII used in CapraFlex™ comes from free-ranged chickens; free of growth hormones, antibiotics, pesticides and insecticides. This form of collagen constitutes a **whole food concentrate** for maximum absorption, and has no known side effects.

Collagen also stimulates production of the cells responsible for maintaining joint-cushioning cartilage. Studies, as those published in *Cell and Tissue Research* have demonstrated collagen has a protective effect on articular cartilage. Now, for the first time, cell researchers have been able to prove in a laboratory study that collagen also stimulates cartilage synthesis in cartilage cells.

CapraFlex contains 1200 mg of collagen per serving. It is unique and powerful because of its four synergistically balanced blends that include:

UNDERSTANDING THE *JARGON*
continued from previous page

potential for heavy metal contamination. For this reason, it's imperative that the source of glucosamine is fully absorbable and, most of all, from a natural Whole Food Source.

• *Chondroitin*—What IT IS & What IT DOES

Cartilage contains chondroitin sulfate, believed to function by drawing fluid into the tissue to give it elasticity and slowdown degeneration by protecting it from enzyme destruction. Cartilage alone, containing *no* blood supply, presents a challenge in transporting new material to where it is needed most.

Studies show chondroitin supplementation slows joint degeneration, improves function and eases pain. Nourishing connective tissue and cartilage is essential for cushioning the joints—a type of shock absorber. The body depends on specific nutrients to assist in maintaining healthy cartilage and connective tissue. Research indicates chondroitin sulfates assist the body in ongoing production and repair processes.

Chondroitin sulfate assists in maintaining healthy synovial

continued on the next page

fluid levels—fluid found between joints that keep them well-cushioned and hydrated, assisting the body in its ongoing production and repair process.

It works in synchronicity with vitamin C in the production and stabilization of collagen, the chief fibrous protein component of connective tissue.

• *Cartilage*—What IT IS & What IT DOES

Cartilage is a specialized form of a very dense connective tissue, consisting of cells embedded in a firm, compact ground substance or matrix. It constitutes part of the skeleton, and is found in parts of the nose, ribs, ears, throat, between the vertebrae, and covers the surface of bones.

• *Collagen*—What IT IS & Where IT IS

Collagen is the principle structural protein in cartilage—providing strength, flexibility and joint support. According to recent studies at Harvard University Medical School, Type II® Collagen derived from chicken cartilage works in synchronicity with the immune system. In addition, studies also show

continued on the next page

1. Osteo-Enhancing Blend—predigested and regular goats milk mineral concentrate. This broad array of naturally-occurring minerals assist in maintaining proper chemical balance to keep calcium in solution (fluid)—preventing it from depositing in the joints. Also contains: calcium phosphate, L-carnitine, oat juice (natural silica) and alfalfa juice (free of gluten).

2. Joint and Cartilage Matrix Blend—contains free-ranged chicken collagen type II, the principal structural protein in cartilage that provides strengths, flexibility and support. In addition, it contains Lutein and a bio-activated green blend of barley, wheat, oat and alfalfa juices (all gluten-free). This blend is predigested and contains 14 strains of beneficial microorganisms and active enzymes.

3. ArthriFlex Blend—contains powerful ingredients known for their strong anti-inflammatory and analgesic (pain reducing) effects, alkalizing effects and anti-oxidants; these include cherry juice, ginger, turmeric, acerola cherry, feverfew, valerian, lemon powder and white willow bark (natural aspirin).

4. Anti-inflammatory Blend—
- Protease blend
- Bromelain
- Papain
- Amylase
- Lipase
- Cellulase

Solution: A complete, comprehensive bone, joint, pain and inflammation reducing support formula. CapraFlex not only fulfills the requirements previously discussed, it also contains cartilage and bone-building ingredients to manage pain, while assisting with damage repair caused by disorders and injuries such as:

- Arthritis
- Fibromyalgia
- Carpal tunnel
- Rheumatism
- Osteoporosis
- Tennis elbow
- Bone-replacement surgery
- Torn/stressed tendons and ligaments
- Rotator cuff injuries

Why Include Goat-Milk Whey for Pain, Inflammation & Injuries?

Because goat-milk mineral whey has been used for decades to promote bone density as well as relieve aching painful joints. This highly concentrated food contains a broad array of naturally occurring minerals (sodium, potassium and calcium) in forms and ratios that are easily absorbed by the body. It contains more than twenty naturally-occurring minerals to assist in maintaining proper chemical balance. An acidic body is associated with bone loss, low bone density and high acid wastes—goat-milk whey has an *alkalizing effect* and neutralizes acid wastes.

Whey *Matters*

In addition to containing more than 20 naturally occurring minerals, necessary for peak performance (mentally and physically), goat-milk whey contains healthy amounts of sodium to control the acid-alkaline balances, equally essential for healthy muscles and bones.

Not Simply A Matter of Calcium

We now know bone health is not simply a matter of taking calcium, it's much more complex.

The mineral combination must be in a form that is used with ease for even the most compromised digestive systems and also be bio-available (easily absorbed).

Research confirms that the standard American diet, high in meat and low in alkalizing fruits and vegetables, leaves an acid residue in the body. It is, therefore, essential that our supplement for bone and joint health, as well as for pain and inflammation, be from a whole-food source such as goat-milk whey, naturally.

UNDERSTANDING THE *JARGON*
continued from previous page

this type of collagen promotes healthy joints and improves mobility and flexibility. Type II chicken collagen is used in the unique product known as CapraFlex™. This type of collagen is naturally accepted for absorption in the body because it recognizes the molecular structure as a whole food. This type of collagen, maintains its integrity and molecular configuration; meaning the molecule hasn't been altered through chemical processing or high temperatures.

• *The Role of Calcium*

We know the importance of calcium to bone health. What we don't often understand is that without the correct balance of minerals, the calcium is either not absorbed, or is stored in unhealthy amounts in various organs— possibly manifesting as bone spurs, or calcium deposits on joints and as kidney stones, to name a few.

Minerals derived from fresh, goat-milk whey are the best source for proper balance. They are essentially pre-digested and, therefore, the body absorbs them like a sponge.

Duration: It's been my experience that CapraFlex should be taken at higher levels for ninety days as directed on the container. Afterward, the amount can be reduced for long-term maintenance after pain and inflammation are managed or eliminated.

CapraFlex™ comes in a powder (easily mixed with protein drinks, non-acidic juices or in a fruit sauce like applesauce). It is also available in easy-to-swallow capsules.

PHYTER #3: CLEAR THE WAY FOR NATURAL REPAIR PROCESSES

Challenge: Reduce inflammation and speed up immunity by producing a cleansing effect that helps to break up circulating immune complexes (CICs) at the center of the body's immune/inflammation reaction. The repair of a disturbed or compromised immune system, however, requires patience and time. You didn't get this way overnight; this book deals with the underlying causes, that takes time.

Systemic oral enzymes stimulate healthy production of messenger immune cells (cytokines). Realistically, following the recommendations in this book, most individuals can expect significant relief within twelve weeks.

Goal: To eliminate the causes, not to suppress or mask the symptoms. Systemic enzyme therapy markedly reduces the body's inflammation level, enabling the person to once again resume normal activity and restore quality of life. If you're in acute pain, your nutritionally-aware physician or healthcare professional can assist you in incorporating prescription drugs (for immediate relief), with systemic enzyme therapy (for long-term repair and maintenance), naturally.

Duration: The effects of systemic oral enzyme therapy on the immune system and treatment of autoimmune diseases, especially rheumatoid factors, are profound, and may involve intense therapy for weeks or months.

After reviewing hundreds of pages on systemic oral enzymes and using several dozen brands, there is only one that eliminated my chronic muscle pain and inflammation during my personal struggle, that is Wobenzym®N. It is manufactured in Germany by the Mucos Pharma GmbH & Co. Wobenzym N is the world's most researched enzyme formula, with over fifty clinical studies supporting its use.

The proteolytic enzymes in Wobenzym N help to break up and destroy bad proteins of CICs, clearing the way for the body's natural repair processes. Studies show Wobenzym N helps to reduce the stiffness and swelling of inflamed joints, increases mobility, and slows further damage.

In Germany it remains a best-selling product, preferred by millions of Europeans over drug therapy and taken daily to maintain good health. I continue to use this product as needed, and continue to see the astounding benefits for both my clients and me.

Sadly, most U.S. health-care providers do not know about systemic oral enzymes. In our conventional medical system, attention is only given to those products studied in the U.S. Most European studies are not totally validated as a basis for clinical opinion in the U.S. Sadly, U.S. medical institutions tend *not* to teach nutrition and non-drug options; they merely teach the bare basics about the use of vitamin and mineral therapies.

Heart Attacks, Stroke & Anti-aging Matter

Wobenzym N has the ability to also help you live longer and healthier. According to world-renowned cardiac specialist Garry Gordon, M.D., "If we can harmonize and re-balance patients' inflammatory pathways, particularly levels of C-reactive protein, we can help them to reduce their risk of heart attacks and stroke. Today, we finally have a safe anti-inflammatory tool: systemic oral enzymes. In my own practice, I emphasize the use of Wobenzym N over aspirin and have had great results in keeping my patients alive and free from heart attacks and stroke, without the concomitant risk of ulcers and hemorrhagic stroke."

Most American medical journals have, until recently, avoided articles on nutrition, feeling they should be published elsewhere (in other countries or health-food-store-type publications). Apparently, a great majority of doctors are uncomfortable recommending a food or natural substance in lieu of drugs. This position has finally begun to change, thanks to physicians who understand and incorporate integrated medicine, combining the best of traditional medical wisdom and conventional medical science.

Wobenzym N are small round tablets, easy to swallow and resemble the famous candy that "melts in your mouth, not in your hand®," except Wobenzym N does not contain artificial coloring. My clients call them their "M & Ns: *medicinal, nutraceutical candy.*"

In my personal and professional experience, systemic oral enzymes offer the first long-term treatment option for inflammatory disorders, with proven healing and safety. This is particularly true when compared to corticosteroids and non-steroidal anti-inflammatory drugs (NSAIDs) with their side effects, of which I'm a prime example.

The results with Wobenzym N are the same as when I took the NSAIDs that almost killed me. At times of acute pain I took ten Wobenzym , three times a day on an empty stomach. As the pain and inflammation subsided, I reduced the dose to five tablets, three times a day. Eventually, as my body healed, I reduced the dose to three tablets, three times a day. Now, I take three twice a day for the health benefits listed, and increase dosage only if I do something that strains my previously injured arm and leg.

Additional Benefits of Wobenzym N— Systemic Oral Enzymes

- **Supports healthy blood flow**—Systemic enzymes help break down the CICs and other dead (necrotic) matter that accumulate in the blood and blood vessels. The body also uses enzymes to regulate the amount of fibrin in the blood, breaking down excess fibrin when the blood becomes too thick. With age, many people do not have enough systemic enzymes; Wobenzym N supports the body's natural blood-thinning processes.
- **Mobilizes the immune system**—Systemic enzymes clean the Fc receptors used by white blood cells to carry away invading pathogens. They also activate the body's second line of defense; the macrophages that remove damaged cells. When damaged cells are not removed, they interfere with the body's normal repair processes.

- **Speeds injury recovery**—After an injury, the body uses large amount of enzymes to facilitate repair. Even young, healthy individuals may experience a shortage of enzymes after injuring a muscle or ligament. This shortage delays the repair process needlessly. Wobenzym N efficiently enhances the body's ability to recover from sprains and strains.
- **Supports tissue cleansing.**
- **Promotes circulation.**
- **Stimulates formation of new healthy tissue.**
- **Increases flexibility of red blood cells**— improving their ability to pass through the capillaries.
- **Activates white blood cells (macrophages)**—the body's natural killer cells, allowing the immune system to deal with inflammation by cleansing itself of cellular debris and quickly neutralizing errant cancer cells.
- **Degrades protein molecules** that penetrate from blood capillaries into the tissues, subsequently causing edema (fluid retention) and exacerbating the inflammatory process.

As we get older, we need more enzymes. This explains why we don't recover as quickly from injuries or illnesses as we age. Our joints no longer repair themselves properly, leading to diseases like osteoarthritis and, additionally, blood begins to thicken, causing disorders of the heart and vascular system, including DVT.

The body performs millions of chemical reactions each second. Most of these reactions need enzymes; the same way a fire needs oxygen to continue burning. Therefore, in order for the body's healing actions to be supported, systemic oral enzymes are a necessary part of any routine for healing and sustaining wellness.

FYI:
- ✔ **Take systemic enzymes on an empty stomach, 30 to 45 minutes before or after a meal.**
- ✔ Wobenzym N can be taken concurrently with any nutritional supplement or medication except for the Warfarin® based blood thinners such as Coumadin™.
- ✔ For daily health maintenance, take three tablets two times a day.
- ✔ For acute injuries, pain and inflammation, take ten tablets three times a day.
- ✔ Before engaging in physically demanding tasks and sports, take systemic enzymes as a preventive measure.
- ✔ If you're already using NSAIDs such as ibuprofen, gradually adjust the dosage over several weeks, follow recommendations of your health care professional.
- ✔ Enzymes are not painkillers and are slower acting than drugs such as aspirin or ibuprofen. You should use Wobenzym N for several weeks, preferably a minimum consistent dose for ninety days before rendering a verdict regarding their effectiveness.

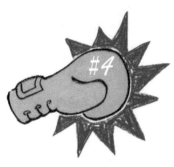

Phyter #4: Tart is Smart®

"TAKE 2OZ. OF TART CHERRY JUICE AND CALL ME IN THE MORNING"

Okay, I know it sounds like this time I've gone over the edge...just stay with me a bit longer, it's you that's in pain, that's why you've read this far. I've already recovered and continue to maintain my health—tart cherry juice is just another part of the overall non-drug recovery protocol that this book aims to share with you.

Tart Cherry Juice, an ancient remedy for gout, arthritis and inflammatory disorders breaks down uric acid crystals that deposit in joints, tendons, kidneys and connective tissue—where it causes inflammation, pain and damage. *Newsweek* magazine even ran an article about its health benefits stating, "Take 10 cherries and call me in the morning."

Recent research confirms tart cherries are a rich source of antioxidants that even assist in the battle over cancer and heart disease. The discovery of the health benefits of tart cherries is part of a larger awareness of the role diet plays in our health, specifically foods known as "functional foods" that offer specific health benefits.

Anti-inflammatory Properties

Daily consumption of tart cherries has the potential to reduce the pain associated with inflammation, arthritis, fibromyalgia and gout. Many middle-aged and elderly consumers are choosing to drink cherry juice rather than take over-the-counter medications to stave off their pains.

"Twenty cherries provide 25 milligrams of anthocyanins, which help to shut down the enzymes that cause tissue inflammation in the first place, preventing and treating many kinds of pain," says Muraleedharan Nair, the lead researcher on

Cherry *Matters*

Tart cherries contain natural anti-inflammatory compounds. In laboratory tests, MSU research indicates that **tart cherry compounds are at least 10 times more active than aspirin**, without any of the adverse side effects.

Research also revealed that the production of a hormone (prostaglandin) is the cause of joint pain. The production of this hormone is directly related to two enzymes. The tart cherry anti-inflammatory compounds are suspected to have the ability to inhibit the enzymes that ultimately cause joint pain.

the cherry project at Michigan State University (MSU). The anthocyanins also may protect artery walls from the damage that leads to plaque build up and heart disease. In fact, the latest research shows that anthocyanins do a better job of protecting arteries than vitamins C and E.

According to research at MSU, tart cherries are an excellent source of compounds with anti-oxidant and anti-inflammatory properties. Anti-oxidants are generally recognized as useful in preventing cancer and other diseases. The anti-oxidant activity of the tart cherry compounds, under the MSU evaluation system, is superior when compared to vitamin E, vitamin C and some other synthetic anti-oxidants.

ANTIQUE ANTIDOTES, MODERN RESULTS

The MSU research, which is still ongoing, substantiates what some consumers have believed for years—tart cherries have important health benefits. In addition, a recent survey of cherry growers shows they have a lower incidence of cancer and heart conditions than the general public. The growers, on average, eat about six pounds of tart cherries per year, while other Americans eat about one pound annually.

Thousands of sufferers are reporting relief since they started a regimen of 2 to 4 oz. of concentrated tart cherry juice a day. Medical doctors and researchers around the country have now concurred that the effectiveness of tart cherries is more than just folklore.

Cherry *Matters*

Cherries have been a popular food for centuries, and now research has demonstrated an amazing array of health benefits derived from a diet that includes tart cherries

According to ongoing research, cherries are a rich source of anti-oxidants that can help fight cancer and heart disease. In addition, they contain compounds that help relieve the pain of arthritis, gout and even headaches.

Research cited to the left was provided by the Cherry Marketing Institute from research conducted by the National Safety and Toxicology Center at Michigan State University;

Strange Name, Powerful Pain Stimulant

Researchers analyzed the ability of the fruits to inhibit cyclooxygenase and act as antioxidants to destroy free radicals. The researchers then quantified the anthocyanin levels of tart and sweet cherries, raspberries, strawberries, blackberries, blueberries, cranberries, elderberries and bilberries.

Cyclooxygenase is produced in the body in two or more forms, termed COX-1 and COX-2, for different purposes. COX-1 is built in many different cells to create prostaglandins, which are used for basic "housekeeping" messages throughout the body. The second enzyme, COX-2, is built only in special cells and is used for signaling pain and inflammation.

Some pain relief medications work by blocking the messages carried by COX-1, COX-2, or both, and thus the body does not feel pain or inflammation. The anthocyanins that are able to block COX-1 and COX-2 are called Anthocyanins 1 and 2, respectively.

Researchers discovered that the antioxidant activity of anthocyanins from cherries was superior to vitamin E at a test concentration of 125 µg/ml. The COX inhibitory activities of anthocyanins from cherries were comparable to those of ibuprofen and naproxen at 10 µM concentrations.

Fresh blackberries and strawberries contained only anthocyanin 2 at a total level of 22.5 and 18.2 mg/100 g, respectively; whereas anthocyanins 1 and 2 were not found in bilberries, blueberries, cranberries or elderberries.

Cyclooxygenase (noun)
cy'-clo-ox'y'gen'ase

Anthocyanins 1 and 2 are present in both cherries and raspberries. The yields of pure Anthocyanins 1 and 2 in 100 g of cherries and raspberries were the highest of the fruits tested at 26.5 and 24 mg, respectively.

TART TASTE, SWEET BENEFITS
The Secret Within

The secret is in the pigments that give cherries their rich red hue. They belong to a class of natural dyes called anthocyanins. These compounds are being called "Mother Nature's all-natural chemo-therapy agents."

In addition to the antioxidants, tart cherries are rich in two important flavonoids—isoqueritrin and queritrin. According to leading researchers, queritrin is one of the most potent anticancer agents ever discovered. Consuming it in foods, such as from tart cherries, is like unleashing an entire army inside your body (James Bond-type agent) who are adept at neutralizing cancer-causing agents.

Antioxidants

Tart cherries are an excellent source of antioxidant compounds. Antioxidants are recognized as useful in prevention of cancer, cardiovascular disease and other illnesses. They may also slow the aging process.

"Eat Your Colors"

Many of us have long suspected a deeper purpose—and a greater genius—encoded in nature's paint box. Now there is research to prove that the brilliant colors of fruits and vegetables are themselves powerful nutrients, and they attract us for good reason.

Perillyl Alcohol and Cancer

Research at the University of Iowa shows that tart cherries contain perillyl alcohol (POH), a natural compound that is extremely powerful in reducing the incidence of all types of cancer. In the

"Tart cherries, specifically
the Montmorency variety,
contain an extremely
significant quantity of
melatonin, enough to
produce positive results in
the body," says Dr. Reiter.

study, perillyl alcohol was found to be up to five
times more potent than the other known cancer-
reducing compounds at inducing tumor regression.

Melatonin Connection

Melatonin has been definitively shown to have
significant anti-inflammatory, antioxidant, and
anticancer properties, as well as improving natural
sleep patterns. Research at the University of Texas by
world-renowned melatonin expert Dr. Russel J.
Reiter, demonstrated that Montmorency tart cherries
contain exceptionally high levels of melatonin, and
in the form most readily utilized by the body.

Dr. Reiter has been painstakingly unlocking the
secrets of melatonin for over thirty years.
Investigations into the role melatonin plays in
organisms and how it is produced has led to many
startling discoveries. Apparently all organisms use
melatonin and it influences a wide variety of
processes in the body.

It now appears that there is a strong link between
diseases, particularly those associated with aging, and
melatonin. This could prove to be one of the most
revolutionary discoveries in the fields of nutrition,
gerontology and a host of degenerative diseases.

Sleep Deprived? Count Cherries Instead of Sheep.

Melatonin, a hormone known for helping to
regulate the body's internal clock, may also help
lower high blood pressure, Dutch and U.S.
researchers reported. Supplements of the hormone,
often used to help battle jet lag, reduced blood
pressure in a small group of men who took them
regularly. The researchers gave melatonin
supplements or placebos to sixteen men with
untreated high blood pressure an hour before they
went to bed. The men who got nightly melatonin
supplements for three weeks lowered their
nighttime systolic blood pressure—the top

number—by about 6 millimeters of mercury on average and their diastolic reading—the bottom number—by 4 millimeters of mercury.

Melatonin, a derivative of an essential amino acid, tryptophan, was first identified in bovine pineal tissue and subsequently it has been portrayed exclusively as a hormone—recently accumulated evidence has challenged this concept. Melatonin is present in the earliest life forms and is found in all organisms including bacteria, algae, fungi, plants, insects, and vertebrates including humans. Several characteristics of melatonin distinguish it from a classic hormone such as its direct, non-receptor-mediated free radical scavenging activity. As melatonin is also ingested in foodstuffs such as vegetables, fruits, rice, wheat and herbal medicines, from the nutritional point of view, melatonin can also be classified as a vitamin. It seems likely that melatonin initially evolved as an antioxidant, becoming a vitamin in the food chain, and in multicellular organisms, where it is produced, has acquired autacoid, paracoid and hormonal properties.

"We were surprised at how much melatonin was in cherries, specifically the Montmorency variety," says Dr. Reiter. The only other fruits that have been examined to date are bananas and pineapples, and both have comparatively low melatonin levels. "Cherry juice concentrate, which involves greatly reducing the water content, has ten times the melatonin of the raw fruit."

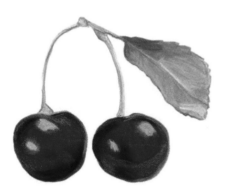

See Resource Section for supplier of Montmorency Tart Cherry Juice Concentrate.

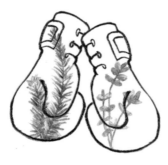

Additional Phyters

The following are what I call "Natures Phyters," mainly because they include various forms of Phytonutrients, ingredients naturally found in nature, that help us win our battle from life-altering disorders:

DL Phenylalanine (DLPA)—contains putative antidepressant and analgesic properties. Pain reduction may occur by limiting enkephalin degradation by the enzyme carboxypeptidase A. The LPA portion acts as a precursor to the synthesis of norepinephrine and dopamine. Note: Do not take when taking nonselective MAO inhibitors.

Boswellia—used in traditional Indian medicine for chronic rheumatic inflammation. Boswellic acids show inhibition of the 5-lipoxygenase enzyme in leukotriene biosynthesis.

Curcumin—the yellow pigment from the Curcuma longa plant that has been used for centuries to treat sprains and inflammation. Studies show it inhibits leukotriene synthesis, platelet aggregation, neutrophil inflammatory response and blocks activation NF Kappa B and promotes fibrinolysis. It was as effective as cortisone or phenylbutazone in acute inflammation.

Bromelain—proven effectiveness in over 400 scientific studies for reducing inflammation and preventing swelling after trauma or surgery. Note: It may enhance the anticoagulant activity of such drugs as warfarin and aspirin.

White Willow Bark—known as "natural aspirin," traditionally used to treat pain because of its salicin content, the precursor to salicylic acid found in conventional aspirin.

Guggal—used traditionally for inflammation of the mouth and pharynx, more recently acclaimed for generalized chronic inflammatory disorders.

Bioflavonoids—shown to possess antioxidant, anti-inflammatory, vasoprotective actions, and anti-allergic mediators through inhibiting histamine release.

Ginger—inhibits platelet thromboxane formation and inflammatory prostaglandin production. Studies show 100% relief from pain and swelling in a small control group.

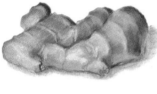

Rosemary—traditionally used for muscular rheumatism and its antioxidant actions.

Papain, Trypsin and Alpha Chymotrypsin—a family of proteolytic enzymes known to speed healing from trauma and injury, as well as reduce edema and inflammation.

Recommended Product—PainX™, a professional product, was formulated with all the ingredients listed above. Suggested dose is one to two capsules without food three times per day. *See resource guide.*

Let the Pain & Inflammation Phyte Start, Naturally!

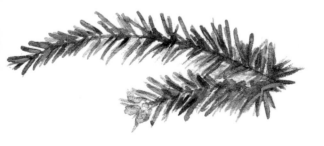

Afterword

PAINFUL REFLECTIONS— HOPEFUL TOMORROWS

When you cause change, you lead.

When you accept change, you regain quality of life.

When you resist change, you stay in the status quo.

It's your pain. It's your decision.

– Dr. Gloria Gilbère

Pain, to the observer, is simply a name for an invisible "something." When the onlooker questions the legitimacy of that something, it's the final blow to the one suffering.

Pain, will never change unless the energy expended to hold onto it is diverted into proven solutions to conquer the fear involved in letting it go.

Pain, particularly when chronic, changes a life forever, sometimes in an instant, others as a slow decline; nonetheless, a way of life transformed at too high a price.

Pain, in a strange way, is a blessing. It helps its victim discover, or often forces its victim to acknowledge, who's there for them, and who's not.

Pain forces us to recognize that "things" don't change, we do; when you're done changing, you're eternally done!

Pain, and the non-drug remedies and subsequent successes, remind us that sustained health is a journey, not a quick-fix destination.

Pain, and the management of it, shall not bend its victim out of shape if the consciousness remains flexible to no-drug options.

Recipe Index

Abbreviated List of References

Ahmed, A.J. "C-Reactive Protein: A Coronary Trojan Horse," *Total Health* (1999). Vol 22, No. 2.

Ahmed, A. J. "The Cycle of Life: Circulation and The Lymphatic System," Manuscript in Preparation (2002).

Department of Cellular and Structural Biology, The University of Texas Health Science Center at San Antonio, San Antonio, TX, USA; Institute of Zoology and Anthropology, University of Gottingen, Gottingen, Germany.

Department of Horticulture and National Food Safety and Toxicology Center, Michigan State University, East Lansing 48824, USA. "The bioactive anthocyanins present in tart cherries," Prunus cerasus L. (Rosaceae) cv.

Fuster, V. *The Vulnerable Plaque: Understanding, Identification and Modification*, (1999). Futura Publishing Co., Inc, Armonk, New York.

Galland, L. *The Four Pillars of Healing*. New York: Random House, 1997.

Hansen, A.A. *Two fatal cases of humans to potato poisoning*. Sci. 61:340.1925.

Holt S, *The Natural Way to a Healthy Heart*, M. Evans and Company Inc, NY, NY. 1999.

HSR Health Supplement Retailer, December 2004:18-19.

In process; Tan DX, Manchester LC, Hardeland R, Lopez-Burillo S, Mayo JC, Sainz RM, Reiter RJ.

Leeds, A. R. 2002. "Glycemic index and heart disease." *American Journal of Clinical Nutrition* 76:286S-289S.

Letteria, J. and Roberts, A. "Regulation of Immune Responses by TGF-b," *Ann. Rev. Immunol.* (1998). Vol. 16 p. 137.

Liu S, Manson JE, Buring HE, et al. "Relation between a diet with a high glycemic load and plasma concentrations of high-sensitivity C-reactive protein in middle-aged women." *American Journal of Clinical Nutrition*, 2002:75:492-498

Liu, S., J.E. Manson, J.E. Buring, M.J. Stampfer, W.C. Willett, and P.M. Ridker, 2002. "Relation between a diet with a high glycemic load and plasma concentrations of high-sensitivity C-reactive protein in middle-aged women." *American Journal of Clinical Nutrition* 75:492-498.

"Melatonin: a hormone, a tissue factor, an autocoid, a paracoid, and an antioxidant vitamin."

MSU Cherry Research Abstract: "Cyclooxygenase inhibitory and antioxidant cyanidin glycosides in cherries and berries." 2001 Sept; Seeram NP, Momin RA, Nair MG, Bourquin LD.

National Federation of Cooperatives Natto: "A Historical Record of Natto," Natto Research Center, Tokyo, Japan, 1977.

Ohkuro, I., Komatsuzaki, T., Kuriyama, S., and Kawashima, M., "The Level of Serum Lysozyme Activity in Animals Fed a Diet Containing Natto Vacilli," Med. Biol. (Japan), 102, 335, 1981.

Rothchild, Bruce. "Fibromyalgia: An explanation for the aches and pains of the nineties." *Comprehensive Therapy*. 17 (1991): 9-14

Rowan, A. and Buttle, D., "Pineapple Cysteine Endppetidases," *Methods Enzymol.*: 244, 555, 1994.

Salvemini, D., Wang, Z., Zweir, J., Samouilov, A., Macarthur, H., Misko, T. Currie, M., Cuzzosrea, J., Sikorski, J, and Riley, D., "A Nonpeptidyl Mimic of Superoxide Dismutase with Therapeutic Activity in Rats," *Science*: 286, 304, 1999.

Seeram NP, Momin RA, Nair MG, Bourquin LD. 2001. "Cyclooxygenase inhibitory and antioxidant cyanidin glycosides in cherries and berries." *Phytomedicine*. Sep;8(5):362–9.

Sumi, H., Hamada, H., Nakanishi, K. and Hiratani, H., "Enhancement of the Fibrinolytic Activity in Plasma by Oral Administration Nattokinase: Natto VR 501," *Acta Haematologica*: 84, 139, 1994.

This book is provided for
educational and informational
purposes. It is not intended to
diagnose, treat, or cure a
disease or condition. For
medical conditions seek the
counsel of a health care
professional. The publisher and
author are not responsible for
the use, effectiveness, or safety
of procedures or products
mentioned.

Published by Lucky Press, LLC
126 S. Maple St.
Lancaster, OH 43130
www.luckpress.com
Order fax: 740-689-2951
Order online at:
www.luckypress.com/gilbere

ISBN: 0-9760576-4-6
Library of Congress
Cataloging Number:
2005922629
Printed in the USA

Illustrations:
    Bonnie Lambert–pastels
    Janice Phelps–watercolors
Food Recipe Development
and Testing:
    Gloria Gilbère
    Ann O'Sullivan
Recipe Editing:
    Paz Hargrave
Editing:
    Janice Phelps
Book Design:
    Bonnie Lambert

Product Resources

Ordering Referenced Products—For your convenience, the professional products mentioned in this book may be ordered toll-free directly from DoctorsChoice, Naturally: 1-866-698-1581 (7:30 to 3:00 Pacific Time M-F), or order online at: www.doctorschoicenaturally.com. This dispensary represents all the products used and recommended by Dr. Gilbère.

Ordering Non-toxic General Merchandise—For an expansive variety of quality air/water purification systems, personal care products, supplements, domestics and books, contact Nutritional Ecological & Environmental Delivery Systems (NEEDS) in the USA at 1-800-634-1380.

Ordering Montmorency Tart Cherry Juice Concentrate *King Orchards*—Direct from the orchard to your door. 1-877-937-5464 or order online at www.mi-cherries.com

Contacting Dr. Gilbère—For information regarding a telephone or in-office consultation, interviews, radio and T.V. shows or general business affairs contact:
- Business Office: (360) 352-3646 (7:30 to 3:00 Pacific Time M-F)
- Fax: (208) 265-1777
- Email: info@drgloriagilbere.com
- Website: www.drgloriagilbere.com
- Mail: P.O. Box 1565, Sandpoint, Idaho 83864 USA